Fighting Pain
Finding Joy

What chronic pain
And 130+ children
Have taught me about joy

By

David Alan Gray

All stories in this book are true. To protect the privacy of those whose stories are shared in this book, names have been changed.

Other books by David Alan Gray
There's Always Time

David Alan Gray

Setting Me Apart

True happiness isn't attained through self-gratification, but through fidelity to a worthy purpose. (Helen Keller)

If you asked me what sets me apart from others, I'd answer, I've had more than 130 children and pain has been my constant companion for many years. I might also argue it's my good looks, my immense intellect and my humility.

Unfortunately, this second statement is subjective, while the first one is 100% true and not subjective at all. I've been blessed with more than 130 children and cursed with constant pain. My wife is my constant companion, and she doesn't like the idea of sharing. Unfortunately, mind-bending pain over my whole body doesn't care. I live with it 24 hours a day, 7 days a week, 52 weeks a year, 60 seconds a minute, and 60 minutes an hour. I think that covers it all. Hang on, there are also 10 years a decade, 10 decades a century and 10 centuries a millennium, except I doubt I'll live 10 decades or 10 centuries and the pain hasn't lasted my whole life. I have no intention of answering whether others think I've been a pain all my life.

To help you understand the concept of full body pain, come with me to a Black Sea resort called Sunny Beach in Bulgaria, Eastern Europe. The local name is Slanchev Bryag, Bulgarian for Sunny Beach. The resort has dozens of hotels close to a beach on the edge of the Black Sea.

Imagine a hot sunny day, and you're on the beach. Visualize yourself looking the best you've ever done and that you're with your spouse, or significant other and they look the best they ever have. I'm sorry if you're picturing a pair of babies on the beach.

There are many other holidaying sunbathers, all in swimsuits. Except, for one young couple, fully dressed, under a beach umbrella. The next day, they're still fully dressed, although in shorter clothes.

On the third day, you're intrigued to see them still fully dressed, hidden under the umbrella.

Whenever my wife, Ann and I go on vacation, we make friends with other holidaymakers. A couple, we'll call Ken and Jean, made friends with us and told us the story of the fully clothed sunbathers. I don't know if the story is true, but I can see how it could happen.

Take things slowly.

They were on their honeymoon, and had misinterpreted the instructions to acclimatize and take things slowly when sunbathing. On their fourth day, they decided they were ready and changed into sunbathing gear. These were small pieces of material, leaving nothing to the imagination. They spent the rest of the day sunbathing. That evening, Jean received a frightened phone call from the bride. When she and Ken got to their bedroom, they found the newlyweds were badly sunburned over their entire bodies. Fortunately, people with the necessary ointments and creams helped them, but they spent the rest of their honeymoon fully dressed, under their beach umbrella. The pain will have stayed for some time and made the first few weeks of their marriage difficult.

I suffer as much pain as those honeymooners did, except mine doesn't go away. Theirs eventually did but, not before their honeymoon ended, but sunburn, sooner or later, stops being a problem. I also don't have the body where I could safely wear a thong style bathing suit. Even when I did, I didn't want to.

Credentials

Some people make stories up, either to make a point or to make themselves seem important. I used to do it myself, and then realized my own stories were worth telling. For example, from aged 16, I drove my motor bike to school every day. One school sports day, my bike was completely blocked in by a teacher's car. She'd parked so close; her car touched the bike. The only way to get out was to move the car. The whole school was outside, and I had no idea where to find the teacher. She wasn't around, but a group of my friends was with me. No one knew who owned the car and the assumption the owner was female, came from the chauvinistic idea of, you wouldn't catch a man dead in a small, light French car that, from the side, looked like a wedge of cheese.

The male contingent, wanting to impress the female contingent, decided to pick the car up and move it back a couple of feet. Here we had a group of 17-year-old boys, watched admiringly by several 17-year-old girls, lifting a small car 12 inches off the ground. As the group shuffles back, they find the car is rusty and, with an unsettling creaking sound, the chassis and body separate. The body stays in the boy's hands, while the chassis smashes to the ground. Being 17, and therefore irresponsible, no one considered the enormity of what had happened. The body was gently placed back on the chassis and we all left. In the years since, I've often wondered how the teacher felt. I don't know who she was and there was no report of a car stopping and the body continuing forward, without chassis or driver.

They are all true

Even though this and my other stories may sound unlikely, they're all true and I was involved in them all. As well as knowing the stories are true, I believe it is essential the people making the claim have the right credentials. For example, is it possible I had a motor bike at 17? Was it possible for a group of boys to try to pick a car up and have the body and chassis separate? To both questions, the answer is yes.

When we attend a conference on making money from selling a product, we want the presenter to be knowledgeable and more importantly, know they've made a lot of money selling the product.

If I wanted you to hire me as a computer consultant, I'd give you my resume, showing the projects I've been involved with and the Fortune 500 companies I've worked for.

When we read a non-fiction book, we should know the author's credentials mean they have the right experience to write the book because they are much more believable.

My credentials

I'm not trying to sell anything, other than this book, but I do want to give you my credentials. I'll start with the pain bit; because that hurts the most. Doctors, who treat patients with chronic pain, seem to write most pain management books. They believe this make them experts.

But, what is an expert? For years, people have accused me of being one, both as a computer consultant and as the father of 130+ children. This makes me believe that many "so called experts" are simply that, so called experts. Expert has two syllables – ex and spurt. An **ex** is a has been and a **spurt** is a drip under pressure. How many doctors are still experts, I'll let you decide. Many will probably still want the title.

There are many things I can be an expert in when it comes to pain and its management.

If you want to know what it is like to not like dogs yet have 3 dogs in your home, I can give you a good perspective and talk from experience.

There are many things I have little or no experience in and I claim no ability. For example, I don't know how it feels having 3 cats in the home. 2 yes, but not 3. I don't know what it is like to be super rich, but am willing to try that one, if I ever can.

Broken bones

My credentials for knowing a lot about pain and its management come from having broken a lot of bones. The parts of my body I've suffered trauma in or on, so far in my life, is mind-boggling.

Make sure you're sitting comfortably, so you won't suffer too much boggle because the next two pages have pictures showing the trauma I've suffered over the years.

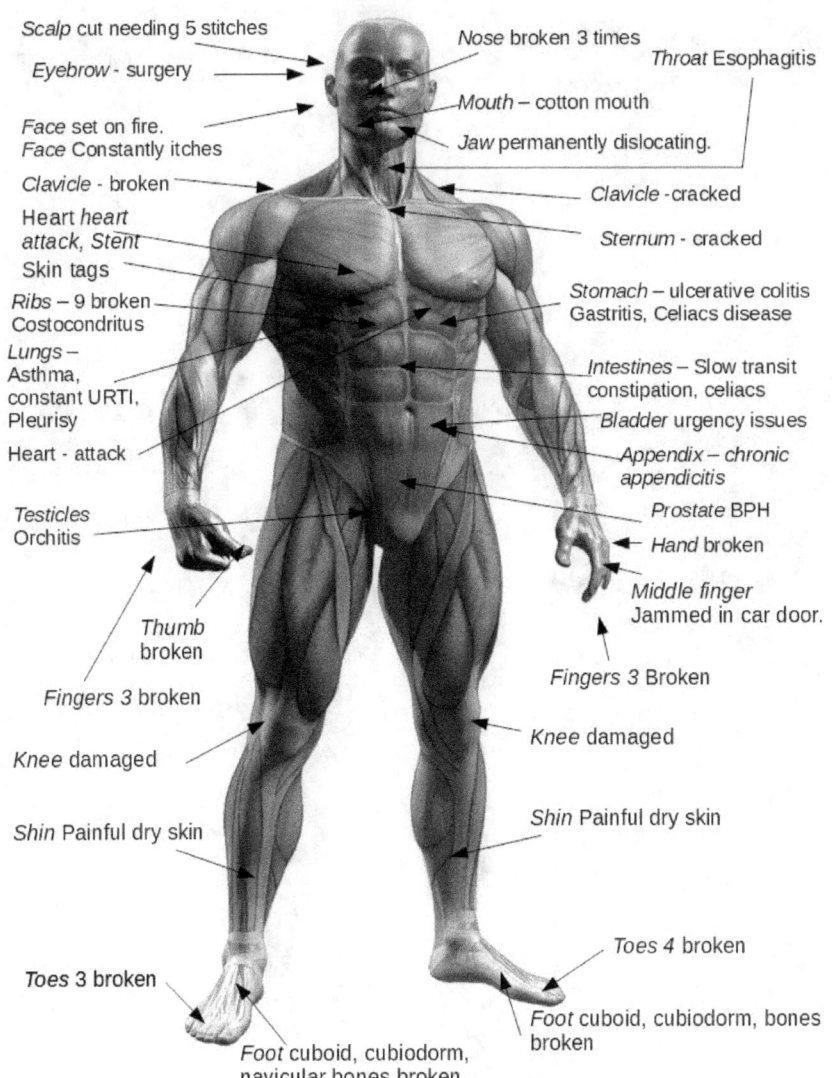

Scalp cut needing 5 stitches

Nose broken 3 times

Throat Esophagitis

Eyebrow - surgery

Mouth – cotton mouth

Face set on fire.
Face Constantly itches

Jaw permanently dislocating.

Clavicle - broken

Clavicle - cracked

Heart *heart
attack, Stent*

Sternum - cracked

Skin tags

Ribs – 9 broken
Costocondritus

Stomach – ulcerative colitis
Gastritis, Celiacs disease

Lungs –
Asthma,
constant URTI,
Pleurisy

Intestines – Slow transit
constipation, celiacs

Bladder urgency issues

Heart - attack

Appendix – chronic
appendicitis

Testicles
Orchitis

Prostate BPH

Hand broken

Thumb
broken

Middle finger
Jammed in car door.

Fingers 3 broken

Fingers 3 Broken

Knee damaged

Knee damaged

Shin Painful dry skin

Shin Painful dry skin

Toes 4 broken

Toes 3 broken

Foot cuboid, cubiodorm, bones
broken

Foot cuboid, cubiodorm,
navicular bones broken

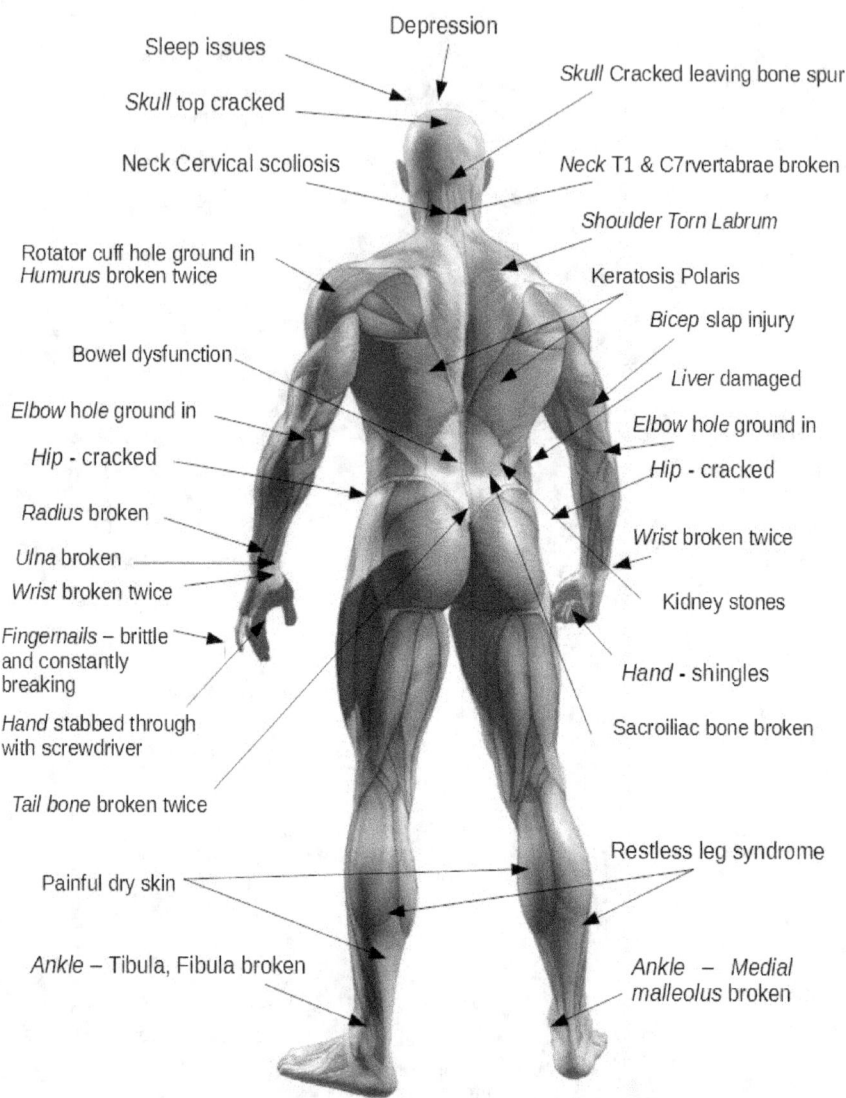

Depression

Sleep issues

Skull top cracked

Neck Cervical scoliosis

Skull Cracked leaving bone spur

Neck T1 & C7rvertabrae broken

Shoulder Torn Labrum

Rotator cuff hole ground in
Humurus broken twice

Keratosis Polaris

Bicep slap injury

Bowel dysfunction

Liver damaged

Elbow hole ground in

Elbow hole ground in

Hip - cracked

Hip - cracked

Radius broken

Wrist broken twice

Ulna broken

Wrist broken twice

Kidney stones

Fingernails – brittle
and constantly
breaking

Hand - shingles

Hand stabbed through
with screwdriver

Sacroiliac bone broken

Tail bone broken twice

Restless leg syndrome

Painful dry skin

Ankle – Tibula, Fibula broken

*Ankle – Medial
malleolus* broken

I've broken 64 bones and suffered trauma in another 41 parts of my body; from head to toe. Some I don't recall exactly how I broke them, but the pain reminds me that I did. I have had over 40 surgical procedures and survived them all.

Taking chances

The world record holder for breaking bones is Robert Craig "Evel" Knievel, a daredevil bike entertainer. He reportedly had 423 bone fractures over his career. I've had several motorbike and car accidents, but am nowhere near his record, nor do I want to be. I've had 70 or so fractures, 1/6th his number. Weirdly, Knievel died from a lung disease.

When younger, I would have enjoyed riding a jet-propelled motorbike over some buses, or the Snake River canyon at Twin Falls, Idaho. I tried the baby step level with jumps over a couple of feet, but nothing like that.

I recently watched several people bridge jumping over the Snake River. A couple offered to let me try. I briefly considered taking them up on the offer, and regretfully had to admit I'm too old and boring. Knievel often didn't clear the obstacles and constantly contributed to his broken bone total.

None of my mishaps has occurred from doing crazy stunts; I guess I'm an unlucky klutz. Some of the stunts **I did do**, were potentially catastrophic and most were definitely crazy. The zaniest was sitting in an inspection channel on a railway bridge, while trains thundered by a foot or less above my head. I'd have lost my head, sitting up slightly too high and given the man who checked the wheels and brakes of each train carriage, an unpleasant surprise. One was a good family friend. I'm glad not to have scarred him for life.

My friends and I would also hang on the bridge's outer ledge. When a train traveled over, we were shaken violently. Talk about having your mind boggled! Losing your grip meant an 8-foot drop to the river below, which, in full flood in the winter, was no deeper than four feet. I didn't hurt myself in any of these adventures. There's a ford a mile or so upstream, with stepping stones. I've fallen off these stones and slipped and fallen on the slippery road surface, but that's the worst. I've abseiled with my son in his wheelchair. I don't mean the son who's in a wheelchair; I mean we tied ropes to him and the wheelchair and abseiled down. I suffered no issues, even though I was under the wheelchair balancing it.

Klutziness– the Gray family ability

Being a klutz seems to run in my family. My father, my sons and at least one grandson are all accidents waiting to happen. One of my "favorites" occurred while I was in bed, asleep. I was dreaming that I was on a railway line and needed to get over a mound of snow because a train was coming. Somehow, I managed to jump sideways over my wife, who insists I didn't touch her, and fell onto the floor on her side of the bed. As I passed by her, she asked me what I was doing. As she did so, I banged my head on her bedside unit, twisted my neck, bit my tongue and hurt my back as I hit the ground. An impossible feat, I'm sure you'll agree. I'm good at it! Another time a friend hit a stick with the front tire of his truck as I was standing nearby. The stick flew about 100 feet in the air and returned to earth arrow like, hitting the top of my foot, breaking a bone or two. Things like this are a common occurrence in my life.

To help me remember I'm a klutz, an evil fairy godmother cursed me with a condition called RSD, when I was 47-years-old. This makes all the damaged parts hurt constantly, as if the trauma just happened. I have no problem calling pity parties, but no one ever shows up.

As a young man, when I'd arrive at a party the host and many others would say, "Hey, here's Dave, what we going to do Dave?" I'd spend the rest of the evening making sure we all had lots of fun. I believe I'd have quickly cleared rooms telling about my mishaps.

130 Children? Not possible!

Before we go any further, let's discuss the number of children Ann and I have had. I can confirm I've been father to over 130

10

children.

No, I'm not a polygamist! I have one wife and she's the mother to the same 130+ children. Having this many children started in 1975, when my family moved 300 miles to the Northeast of England. I was 6,000 miles away in America, at the time, but I found them.

Not long after we met, Ann and I began dating and eventually began to talk about marriage. We wanted a large family and joked we might have enough for our own soccer team. We didn't expect to have enough for an entire league and, were surprised that a few months after our 30th wedding anniversary, our 100th child was born.

An average family?

For the first ten years of our marriage, we were an average family, whatever that means. Our first three children were born in 1978, 1983 and 1986. Life changed in 1991, when our fourth child was born, although we didn't know it at the time. #30 was born in 2001 and #50, confusingly, was born in 2000. #75 was born in 2003 and #100 in 2008; #110 came along in 2009; #115 in 1999; #120 showed up the day before Thanksgiving in 2010, having been born in April. By July 2012, the number had reached 130. You may have guessed Ann and I are foster parents. We have adopted 6 of them.

It's my life, not yours

My life is simply that, my life. What has happened to me, affected me and affected me differently from anyone else. My family was involved in a car accident and we all experienced the accident differently, although it was the same event.

Did you notice the word "different" shows up several times? This isn't accidental, I want to emphasize that we all experience life differently and uniquely. I can share my experiences and tell you how I manage the pain. You can at least try what I have and hopefully find relief.

I've been through so many trials; my friends have given me the nickname Job, as in the Bible. These trials have shown me how to find silver linings in clouds apparently so black, so dense, nothing is visible. This has become the main goal in life, Fighting Pain and Finding Joy.

Who is worst off?

My son was born with Cerebral Palsy and has suffered through many surgeries to help him walk correctly. They all failed. I can't walk without pain. My problems only started in 2008; his when he was born.

In 2013, I was diagnosed with Celiac's disease, which means I must watch what I eat, because gluten makes me sick. My grandson was born allergic to both lactose and casein and must avoid milk products.

Who is worst off? The answer is, both and neither of us. It's an apples and pears type of comparison. Since birth, my son hasn't walked without pain. I know how; I no longer can. My grandson won't know how it feels to eat what everyone else does. I knew until 2010.

We irrationally think we're all the same. We believe our way of thinking and behaving is the right way. When something happens, and we're merely ticked off, we're surprised when someone else gets angry. The reverse is also true, people who go off the deep end, when presented with a situation, can't conceive someone else may only be ticked off, or not even bothered. What bothers us, may, or may not, bother others and even though we know this, it seems inconceivable that this could be possible. If it bothers me, what's wrong with them, that it doesn't bother them?

We are all different

130+ children have proved to me that children all respond differently and are likely to respond differently in the future. Annoyingly, what works with one child in one situation, may not work with the same child in another situation. It seldom works with a different child in any situation. Frustratingly, the same child may well behave differently, in the same situation in the future.

It's impossible to pigeonhole children, except by gender. In our case, we can say 80 have been girls and the rest boys. Unfortunately, this doesn't help us know how a child will behave. We can make general statements about what a boy or a girl will do, but that's it.

Are newborn children blank sheets?

Until recently, most child experts and psychologists believed that, at birth a child was a blank sheet of paper and their development depended on how good or bad a set of parents they had. If you had a difficult child, you were doing something wrong. A badly behaved child had parents too lenient or too strict, depending on which so-called expert you listened to. There seemed to be no end to the problems caused by parents, even when the child was an adult.

These same experts now admit a person is born with a personality. Over half our children came to us as newborns, and each has arrived with a unique personality. We're all born with unique character traits, needs and talents. These traits help us decide how we'll behave and react in any given circumstance.

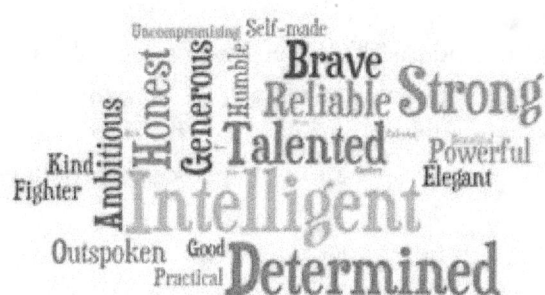

Toys and Joys

I'm sure you realize that as adults we all behave differently, even in the same situations.

Some of us can share our toys; others will scream and shout if we try to take it off them. This happens with children as well.

I still find joy with my computer, even though I can no longer do much of what I used to be able to. My safe place is in front of my computer, writing.

Our character traits decide the way we look at life, how we do what we do and how we handle pain and disappointment. Some of us are timid, nervous and shy; others show courage and firmness. Some grow up to be politicians or lawyers and others grow up to be useful members of society. Some feel uncomfortable when we lie, others delight in being dishonest. This suggests politicians can't help themselves, they were born that way.

Looking back

It wasn't until I was a mature adult and able to look back over my life, that I realized I was born with my set of characteristics, or talents. Some I've improved, others I haven't. I now realize I didn't have the problems and issues I thought I had as a child and young adult. I had a normal upbringing, unless you talk to Ann and she'll tell you I was strange until she came along. She might also argue about my maturity level. I have no control over getting older, which is mandatory. Growing up, however, is optional. I've decided not to exercise my option.

As my purpose in life is to find joy wherever I can, some of what I do seems to embarrass my wife and children, especially my children. I, naturally, do the embarrassing, silly action as many times as I can. This makes me happy and leaves no space to worry about the pain or anything negative.

We may not be consciously aware that what happens to us each day teaches us. Let me rephrase that a little. Every experience we have, whether good or bad, teaches us something. They mold us into the people we are. Unique, exceptional, diverse, distinct human beings, who are hopefully learning from what happens to us.

Didn't know I didn't know that

I've been taught things I didn't realize I wanted to know. I know about handicapped children and how their disabilities can cause difficulties for them and their parents. I know the horror of losing babies in the womb, both to miscarriage and to death in utero. I don't know this in the same way Ann does, but I know how ghastly and distressing it is.

I know the horror of losing a baby we've loved and cherished for several months or years. The fact they left us to go live with family

14

members, is no better than had they died, as we generally don't see them again and when we do, they have no idea who we are.

None of these events has brought me any joy. Losing a baby is a devastating loss that takes a lot of time and effort to process and put behind us. We have lost 60+ babies who came to us as newborns and all left before they were 6-months old. They are gone forever, not dead, but not with us either. We've also lost our other foster children, many of whom were also babies. Each time a child has left they have taken a piece of our heart with them when they left us. We've learned how to deal with the horror and grief this has caused. We have lost children to death in utero and to "normal" death, so we know how horrible it all is.

Spirit Bubble

To do one's best in the face of the commonplace struggles of life—and possibly in the face of failure—and to continue to endure and to persevere in the ongoing difficulties of life when those struggles and tasks contribute to others' progress and happiness and one's own eternal salvation—this is true greatness.
(Howard W Hunter)

We are magnets; we attract the emotions we put out. Imagine there's a bubble all around each of us. Inside this bubble with us, are the emotions, feelings, the pain and happiness, our attitude towards life in general.

We've all suffered through the concept of personal space, if we have been in a car for more than 10 seconds with more than one child in the back. Our spirit bubble is simply an extension of this personal space and like it, is invisible.

Emotions pass back and forth through our bubbles and the spirit bubbles of those we meet. In biology, you may remember hearing about osmosis. Wikipedia has this description, which is meaningless to the layperson.

Osmosis is the spontaneous net movement of solvent molecules through a semi-permeable membrane into a region of higher solute concentration.

In simpler terms, things pass through a membrane, such as a bubble, **to** the side with the higher concentration, **from** the side with the lower concentration.

If we have the attitude, the strong emotion, of being in pain and depressed, we can suck all the positive emotions from someone else's bubble and replace it with our negative emotion. Fortunately, this takes time and only works if the other person's bubble is not chock-full of positive emotions. If their positive emotion is stronger, our negative emotion will bounce off. If it is a lot stronger, they can suck our negative emotions and replace them with their positive ones. I have no control over whether my spirit bubble fills with emotions, it does it automatically.

When I say a spirit bubble, I don't mean a spiritual bubble, which suggests something religious. There's nothing wrong with being religious, but when I say spirit bubble, I mean the place emotions go. We can learn to control which emotions stay in, but if we have an emotion, it automatically goes into our bubble. The photograph of me above, shows me inside my spirit bubble. I cannot see the emotions or my spirit bubble, but I believe it looks something like this and comes with me everywhere I go, even when I'm dressed as wonderfully as I am here.

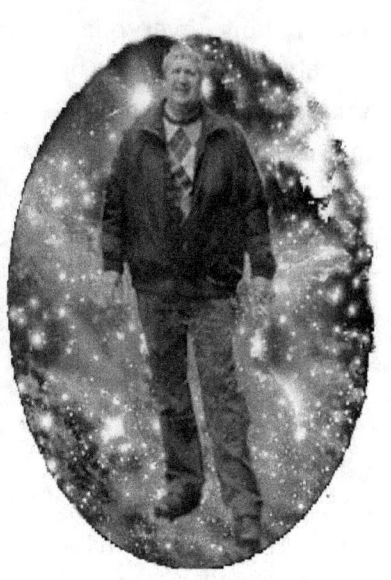

The strongest emotion wins

Let's say we're overwhelmed because we're hurting more than normal, due to the chilly weather. We're tired and miserable because we're not getting enough sleep at night. To round it all out, several members of our immediate family are sick and we need me to nurse them back to health. In other words, we're disgruntled and are purposely filling our spirit bubble with powerful, negative emotions. Our brain's limbic system, which handles emotions, puts us on a heightened level of alert in case we need to fight or run away.

When our highly-charged spirit bubble meets another spirit bubble, there's a battle to decide which has the highest emotion or emotional index if you like. The bubble with the highest index will generally overwhelm the one with the lower index. When negativity wins, the person becomes irritated and displeased for no reason they can figure out.

You will have seen this happen, I'm sure. Someone with a highly negatively charged spirit bubble can suck the joy straight out of a room, making everyone miserable. A person with a powerfully positively charged spirit bubble, full of joy, seems to be able to suck the misery out and replace it with happiness. Which one we are is a choice we can make. I have made the choice of a positively charged bubble, so the negative issues from the areas of my body which hurt can be overwhelmed.

Mirror, mirror.

A lot of research has been done on how to get us to part with our money, especially in restaurants and the most successful is mirroring.

If we're surly, don't be surprised if others are surly. If we want good service in a restaurant, be positive and pleasant to the server. If we want poor service, project surliness and that's what we'll get back. Our spirit bubbles are invisible, but the charge they carry, the emotions inside the bubble are detectable. They show in our body language, our face and voice. Most of us don't have poker faces; even those of us who are good at poker can't always maintain that straight face.

It's impossible to appear to be happy when our voice sounds unhappy. A good example is a server in a restaurant who has the ability to bring us out of our funk. She has learned how to put up barriers to other people's negativity because she knows negatively charged people give little or no tips. Whatever her reasons, it works and we generally give her larger tips.

Where do emotions go?

Our spirit bubbles are permeable and emotions pass through in either direction. So, where do emotions go when we push them out? If we can suck the joy from a room, or suck the misery out, where do they go? To be perfectly honest, I don't know. An Internet search will tell us that emotions warn us about what is happening in our lives. They control our thinking and our behavior and affect our bodies. To keep life interesting, our bodies affect our emotions. The search will also tell us we need to learn how to release the emotions causing us problems. Most searches have returned little detail on how to release our negative emotions, just the need to do so.

There is no literature on where they go. I'm sure they don't litter the places we've been, waiting to mug unsuspecting passers-by. I hope not, because negative emotions fit the concept of releasing them and, if they come back, we know no one else wants them either. Wherever they finish off going, I know we **can** release them, both the useful ones and the useless ones.

Who is in charge?

One weird thing about our spirit bubbles is that the person in charge can vary. It will constantly be us, but sometimes it may be the 7-year-old us. At other times the younger, better looking us we think we still are; or it can be the current version of us.

We were at some hot springs as a family, when one of our girls I hadn't seen for some time, came into the water. Immediately, the teenage me took over. I picked her up and dunked her under the water. I told her about this urge and she unsuccessfully pleaded with me to fight it. Having dunked her, I let go and the adult me took control again.

Go see a doctor

It may feel as if our spirit bubble is chock-full of negative emotions and nothing we do makes a difference. In this case, you may be clinically depressed and it's essential you visit with your doctor.

In many cases, clinical depression can only be resolved with medication. I take lots of medication to combat the pain I suffer. It's essential I take them as prescribed by my doctor. The same is true for you, if you take medications for your pain. Fighting Pain Finding Joy can only work if we do all we can to make sure the pain is under control.

I have been told about many homeopathic remedies. I have tried some, so far, with no success.

I have tried coming off my medications, because they were known to interfere with a new procedure. I have also tried dozens of different pain medications with little or no positive results. I have tried changing medications with dramatic results all in the wrong direction. To date, nothing has worked better than the those prescribed by my doctor.

Manage my emotions

I am left with one option. Manage the emotions that flood into my spirit bubble. Being in a lot of pain means that many, indeed most, of the emotions overflowing into my spirit bubble are negative. Pain always seems to bring harmful feelings and it is a fight to overcome the negativity. If I want to succeed at anything, I have no option but to do all I can to manage those negative emotions and send them to the curb where they can do no harm. I have to be sure the space made is filled with positive emotions. My goal is find joy in everything I do. It is a work in progress because I don't achieve it all day, every day.

Who should I avoid?

I have heard and read experts who suggest that we should avoid people who cannot manage their emotions. They don't use the term spirit bubble, as I invented that term, but they are talking of the same thing.

If a person is capable of sucking the joy out of a room, that same person can suck the joy out of a single person as well. How should we deal with such a person?

One suggestion is that we avoid them totally. Don't give them the chance to negativize you. It is easy to identify people who have negatively charged spirit bubbles by the effect they have on you. So should you avoid them? What if they are your family members, your spouse, your boss?

As we go on I'll answer these questions, but to put it simply, I believe we should be helping them as much as we possibly can, to make their spirit bubbles fill with positive energy. The only people I believe we should be avoiding in this situation are people who are casual acquaintances with powerfully negatively charged bubbles who, unless we make a real effort, will be nothing more than that. Even then, I wonder whether we shouldn't try to help them fight their pain and find joy.

Finding Joy

To get the full value of joy you must have someone to divide it with.
(Mark Twain)

Many of my life experiences have been exciting and given me immense joy. I enjoyed standing in a court, when Ann and I have adopted children, and answering some odd questions, to convince a judge to allow us to adopt a child born to another father and mother. They asked about our willingness and ability to take the child into our home and treat them as a normal child. Even now, I don't know what one of those is, but we answered yes.

Some questions are similar to those we answer on those visa forms we fill out, when we go to another country. The one on the visa form and for adoption is my favorite.

"Have you ever been arrested or convicted for any offense or crime, even though subject of a pardon, amnesty or other similar legal action? Have you ever unlawfully distributed or sold a controlled substance (drug), or been a prostitute or procurer for prostitutes?"

Who would answer yes, even if they were? Nevertheless, the bureaucracy insists it's asked. Having answered the questions correctly, the judge gives advice and instructions on what it meant to be adding another child to your family tree. How we had to had to treat him or her as if we were their birth parents.

They get a new name and birth certificate, with their new name, showing us as their parents. The joy of this is as indescribable as holding a newborn. There are only a few other times when my spirit bubble was so positively charged and full of joy as when I first held my newborn child, or had a judge tell me an older child is now my newest baby and they are now part of our family.

Please wash the dishes

If you're like me, you go out to celebrate. When the check arrives, you ask the waiter to have the newly adopted child escorted to the kitchen, where she should wash dishes to pay the bill. I wish I'd had the presence of mind to have videoed the look on 10-year-old Elizabeth's face, when the waiter returned carrying a silver platter with some rubber gloves and gently pulled her chair back. She had stood up and stepped towards the kitchen, before she realized I was teasing and sat back down complaining about me.

I love this story so much I take every opportunity to retell it. Elizabeth died four weeks later, so it helps to keep her memory fresh and brings me joy. Even though the experience ended with the death of my daughter, remembering February 20, 2002, always makes me happy. My spirit bubble fills with joy and there is little or no room for negative emotions.

Getting older

One joyful phase of life is when a child gets married. We gain a child-in-law and can look forward to being a grandparent. Most of the stress is on the father's wallet. As we want to be different, when our oldest daughter married, our then youngest was 3-years-old. In fact, that daughter's oldest child is three years older than my current youngest child. Four of our grandchildren are older than her, with our oldest grandchild 5 years older. When she graduates from college, I'll be 76. When my youngest biological child graduated, I was a more reasonable 52-years-old.

A 14-year-old girl we know said, "So?", when I told her this, in response to her question about whether we were going to adopt our youngest daughter. I enjoy her answer so much I tell the story as often as I can.

Our children didn't all fly the nest early. They married in reverse age order, so we have constantly had children in our home. I look

23

forward with joy to the day the ones at home get married. My wallet looks forward with fear, at the thought that four are girls all who will want expensive weddings. I tried to convince our oldest daughter to elope with half the money it was going to cost me for the wedding. She refused to even consider the idea.

Men are that they might have joy

Instead of calling pity parties, my goal is to be happy, have joy, and live by the idea **"Men are that they might have joy."** (Book of Mormon 2 Nephi 2:25) This statement has no qualifiers and sounds wonderful. Despite the pain I'm in, I've learned we can decide to be joyful, come what may!

We first need to find out what these women, Joy and May, have to do with managing pain. We can rule out the idea Joy and May are fairy godmothers who, by waving their magic wands, will get rid of all our pain. Let's use the Internet for a definition for joy.

Context and Perspective

A word's meaning can only be understood using context and perspective. My high school French teacher taught this with a joke about a Frenchman learning English.

His language teacher wrote the letters OUGH on a chalkboard and asked the class to pronounce the word. Next, he added letters. B ough is pronounced bow, c ough is pronounced cof, d ough is pronounced doe and on through all the variations, all of which are pronounced differently. The Frenchman spent the next week muttering, b ough is pronounced bow, thr ough is pronounced threw, en ough is pronounced enuf, etc. It took over his life, and he was ecstatic, when he got them all correct at the next class. His elation was short-lived, because as he was sitting on a bus heading to his apartment, he saw a poster reading, "Star Wars is pronounced success."

We'll leave our poor Frenchman crying on his bus, because he doesn't realize the word "pronounced" has multiple meanings. Let's look up the synonyms for joy. The first is pleasure.

The fun oriented person often finds pleasure anywhere. Some people even find pleasure being antisocial. Pleasure is associated with self-indulgence, self-satisfaction and self-gratification. The antonyms, or words with the opposite meaning, include self-denial and abstinence. Did you notice how many times the word 'self' shows up? It seems obvious that selfish fits the definition.

Pleasure

My search for "What is pleasure?" returned a definition of 'a feeling resulting from the satisfaction of a physical, emotional or intellectual need.' Some people find pleasure in social activities, such as reading, music and being outdoors. Many definitions state pleasure is the opposite or absence of pain and pain is the absence of pleasure. I suffer from chronic pain across my whole body, and the idea there's no possibility of joy for me, seems ridiculous, unreasonable, bizarre and unfair. You'll have to use your imagination and visualize me feeling sorry for myself. Chronic pain is defined as persistent severe pain lasting more than 12 weeks, is difficult to treat and shows no likelihood of ever stopping. That is RSD as it affects me. The pain never stops, never gets better and never stops making me upset.

Humor

To help me get over my sulking and find some joy, here is the most ridiculous lawsuit ever filed. In 1991, Richard Overton sued beer company Anheuser-Busch for $10,000. He claimed to have suffered emotional distress, mental injury, and monetary loss when drinking their beer didn't make his fantasies of beautiful women in tropical settings come to life, as he claimed they'd advertised. This drove him to buy and drink more Bud Light. Not too surprisingly, the Judge dismissed the case. Overton expected a lot more pleasure from drinking his beer than he got. He complained, because he found no joy.

To stay with fun, here are a couple of odd statements made on insurance claims.

25

> **"He was all over the road. I had to swerve several times before I hit him."**

My personal favorite claims,

> **"I found that my window was actually up when I put my head through it."**

I'm almost over my sulking, so we'll finish off with some bizarre laws. Did you know it's illegal to put coins in your ears in Hawaii? In Lubbock Texas, you can't sleep in a garbage can. Los Angeles has banned washing two babies, in the same bath, at the same time. Californians can't legally peel an orange in a hotel. In Winchester, MA, you can only walk on a tightrope in church. The weirdest one makes me wonder when someone in Idaho tried to fish for trout, while sitting on a giraffe.

Canada's on-line legal magazine Slaw, reports there's a Canadian law forbidding people from jumping from a plane without a parachute. It would be interesting to know how many people have been prosecuted for that one and what the penalty was.

It's also illegal in Canada to board a plane while it's in flight. So be warned, if you have super powers and can fly, don't board a Canadian plane if it's not on the ground, they may try to arrest you.

Life begins when pain ends

An advert for varicose vein surgery claims life begins when the pain ends, suggesting we can't live any sort of life with pain. This can't be true, because I find pleasure at many times and places, that don't need me to be pain free.

Children love me. I'm not totally sure why, it might have to do with the number I've had. Babies in shopping carts especially love me. This occurs with people of all ages, but with babies I can much more easily interact with them. Recently, one little girl watched me as I walked past. While I was in front of her, she had no problem; as I moved beside her, she only had to turn her head. When I was a few yards away, she couldn't see me, without turning her head in an owl-like manner. As this is impossible, she had a problem, which took her a few seconds to resolve. She turned around and moved her head the other way. This made me laugh. I found joy, even though before, during and afterwards I hurt a lot.

The dictionary says pleasure is the antonym or opposite of pain and therefore the two cannot exist at the same time. So, we have a definition issue. If pleasure is the antithesis of pain, how can I have both enjoyed the moment and been suffering a huge amount of pain? Right now, I'm in pain, and enjoying the thought you're thinking, "Why is he using words like antithesis instead of opposite?" The answer is because I try to inject humor wherever I can. My children have perfected their eye rolling techniques and I love giving them opportunities to do so. I find humor positively charges my spirit bubble and forces any negative emotions out.

Not Superman

I once gave a lot of people pleasure using a public telephone box. Those of us who are baby boomers remember the time before cell phones and smart phones existed. Back before 1985, which my younger children tell me is in prehistory, the only phones available, other than house phones, were public phones. They were everywhere. It was the only way to make phone calls if you were not at home or in an office. I used one in a crowded public place and caused a huge amount of pleasure for a lot of people.

The phone booth was supposed to have glass panels. I didn't realize the glass on the left side was missing and leant against it. There were only two possible scenarios. I'd fall over, or I'd stay balanced sideways, because I'm a superhero with power over gravity. Gravity partially won. The phone wire designer seems to have allowed for such an occurrence. I didn't hit the ground. I was left hanging on the phone, hoping and praying the wire wouldn't break.

Passers by seemed to think my predicament was hilarious, yet no one offered to help. This irritated me but being upset didn't get me upright.

I'm sure all their spirit bubbles were full of pleasure, but mine wasn't, especially because gravity was playing games and making me circle. It took me several minutes to pull myself back up. I then finished off making the phone call I had started.

If giving this sort of fun and pleasure to others is joy, please count me out. I'm not interested in hurting either myself, or anyone else. I don't want my life to be pleasurable based on the idea someone was hurt in some way or another. Especially when it's me getting hurt.

Happiness

So, real joy isn't pleasure and, as fun sounds to me to be the same as pleasure, what's left? Should we join our French friend crying on the bus, because we don't understand the word joy? This next synonym will hopefully help us avoid that fate – happiness. I believe this fits the definition of joy better than any other synonym,

In no order, here are some excellent quotes about happiness.

True happiness isn't attained through self-gratification, but through fidelity to a worthy purpose. *Helen Keller.*

Hope is itself a species of happiness, and, perhaps, the chief happiness, which this world affords. *Samuel Johnson.*

Happiness is man's greatest aim in life. Tranquility and rationality are the cornerstones of happiness. *Epicurus.*

Realize that true happiness lies within you. Waste no time and effort searching for peace and contentment and joy in the world outside. Remember that there is no happiness in having or in getting, but only in giving. Reach out. Share. Smile. Hug. Happiness is a perfume you can't pour on others without getting a few drops on yourself. *Speaker / writer Og Mandien.*

Happiness is contagious... when you reflect happiness, then all others around you catch the happy bug and are happy too. *Author Jennifer Leese*

Happiness is when what you think, what you say, and what you do are in harmony. *Mahatma Gandhi.*

Happiness is an inner state of well-being. A state of well-being enables you to profit from your highest: thoughts, wisdom, intelligence, common sense, emotions, health, and spiritual values in your life. *Lionel Ketchian. President of LRK Communications and the Founder of the Happiness Club.*

A happy person isn't a person in a certain set of circumstances, but rather a person with a certain set of attitudes. *Broadcaster Hugh Downs.*

Happiness is the meaning and the purpose of life, the whole aim and end of human existence. *Aristotle.*

Money can't buy you happiness, but it does bring you a more pleasant form of misery. *British comedian Spike Milligan.*

It isn't easy to find happiness in ourselves and it isn't possible to find it elsewhere. *Essayist Agnes Repplier.*

Happiness is mostly a by-product of doing what makes us feel fulfilled. *Dr. Benjamin Spock.*

Happiness is the only good. The time to be happy is now. The place to be happy is here. The way to be happy is to make others so. *Lawyer and lecturer Robert Green.*

There is work that is work and there is play that is play; there is play that is work and work that is play. And in only one of these lie happiness. *Humorist, Frank Gelett Burgess.*

Happiness for me is to know that my life has meaning and purpose, and that every day my life touches others in a positive way – whether to make them laugh or learn or both at once! *Teacher, coach, and writer Deanna Mascle.*

Happiness is something you get as a by-product in the process of making something else. *Aldous Huxley.*

Whoever is happy will make others happy too. *Mark Twain.*

Happiness can be defined, in part at least, as the fruit of the desire and ability to sacrifice what we want now for what we want eventually. *Author/motivational speaker Stephen Covey.*

This last one, from the ancient Greek philosopher Socrates (born 469BC, died 399BC), is my favorite definitions of a philosopher. I'm

29

not unhappy being married, but I love what it says about being a philosopher.

> By all means, marry: If you get a good wife, you'll become happy; if you get a bad one, you'll become a philosopher.

It fits in well with the joke about what a philosophy major asks on the first day of work after graduating and finding a job where their degree is useful.

Answer "Do you want a soda with your burger?"

Joy is happiness

These quotes and my other research, make me realize the joy in "man is that he might have joy" is happiness. Joyful people find joy and happiness everywhere. They are the ultimate optimists. It is the only word that works for me and makes perfect sense. It's one of those "duh" moments when you think "of course it is".

My Plan of Happiness

To have joy in our lives, we must have a plan. No project is successful without a plan. A plan of joy sounds odd, so as joy is happiness, what we need is a plan of happiness. Something which makes sure our spirit bubbles is positively charged. We do this, or at least I do, by taking every opportunity to find joy.

I found joy one Saturday before Christmas, while waiting for Ann and two of our daughters to come out of a shop, by saying "Merry Christmas" to people passing by. Most people ignored me, but some responded and smiled. The two daughters with me constantly tried to stop me. They failed and even that gave me joy. I was doing it because, trying to bring happiness, a little ray of sunshine into someone else's life, made me happier and brought me joy, even when in pain.

My spirit bubble must release some negative emotions to make room for the joy. This is a big part of my plan of happiness. Replace negative emotions with positive emotions. If our spirit bubble is full of positive emotions there is no room for negative ones. It is impossible to hold both emotions at the same time. You can't be happy and sad at the same time.

Bullying

Some people find ways to be happy without bringing any joy. There are people who enjoy hurting others. This sort of behavior doesn't bring happiness to the other person and therefore, can't be joy. I recently came across a definition for bullying. If someone is accidentally unpleasant to you, that makes him or her rude. If they purposely did it, they're being mean. If they keep on doing it, even after we ask them to stop, they are bullying. The bully may find joy in their behavior and the pain they inflict, but it's one sided. The victim finds no joy.

Lobster danger

Another rule in my plan of happiness is finding joy in the memory of what has happened in the past, even if they weren't necessarily fun when they happened. Reliving / retelling them brings me immense joy.

In 1976, Ann's family invited me to go on holiday with them to Ilfracombe in Devon. We'd been dating for a year by then. Her brother, Kevin, took his friend Chris along and the three of us shared a tent.

One day, we hired a four-man dinghy and set out into the Atlantic Ocean. After about 10 minutes, we came across some lobster pots and pulled them up. By we, I mean me, Kevin and Chris. Ann threatened to get out of the dinghy unless we stopped. We didn't and so she screeched and insisted she'd get out of the dinghy.

Go where?

We were 300 yards from the beach, so couldn't work out where she could go, as we had decided not to wear life jackets. After a few minutes, we stopped mocking her and let the pot wire go. The pot sank to the bottom very quickly and Ann sat down again muttering threats under her breath.

Only then did we notice the incoming tide had pushed us around a headland and we were heading to shore. There was nothing we could do, except get swept onto a steep rocky beach. We realized we needed to get back out to sea and around the headland.

The beach was narrow, with a towering cliff on three sides. We tried running out, but the steepness of the beach and the power of the incoming tide, meant before we could jump in the dinghy; it was already 10 feet up the beach behind us. Kevin put the dinghy on his head and ran out.

The tide took his feet from under him and wrapped the dinghy rope around his neck. He vanished under the water, and both he and the dinghy finished off at the same point on the beach which was now about 8 feet from the water.

Let's climb the cliff

We examine the cliff walls, where someone had cut steps into the cliff wall. As we couldn't get back out to sea, we dragged the dinghy up the cliff. We didn't consider simply sitting in the dinghy, until the tide came in and paddling back out and round the headland. Hindsight is always 20-20!

We walked, in our swimsuits, the 3 miles, back to town, carrying a bright yellow boat, along a narrow country road with no sidewalks and plenty of cars.

Writing this brings me joy and laughter even 40+ years later. My spirit bubble fills with happiness every time I recall this experience. I can only imagine how it looked for the drivers of the cars that went past, but I imagine if they do recall it, they find joy as well. I would love to know what they believed we were doing. I also wonder what on earth we were doing, going on the open sea with no life jackets.

RSD / CRPS

Happiness is man's greatest aim in life.
Tranquility and rationality are the cornerstones of happiness
(Epicurus)

One area of my life that brings me no happiness is the never-ending pain. Unless I have broken yet another bone, I only see doctors for medicine checks.

The last time I was at a pain doctor, we reviewed my list of problems and set levels where 0 out of 10 means no pain and 10 out of 10 is the worst pain ever. We did this for the many areas of my body that hurt and scored them all on the high end. We reviewed all the interventions I'd tried. After about 30 minutes, he concluded there was nothing he could do for me. The only positive from the visit is that he didn't charge me any money for his time.

A different pain clinic doctor had previously told me to expect the pain to get worse and that the RSD would probably spread to other parts of my body.

Say what?

Most people, including many doctors, are confused about this prognosis. In what they consider the normal way it all works, we have a painful event, such as a broken wrist. We have excruciating pain, so we go to hospital and, after x-rays are taken, etc. we sit around, while the doctors and nurses chat and hit on each other. Eventually, someone notices us and puts our wrist in a cast. For the next few weeks, we suffer through the discomfort of having our arm encased. We take pills and try to work out how to manage with the cast on. We go mad from itching and use knitting needle scratchers, hoping to stop the itching, without doing any damage. After several weeks, the bone is checked and, if healed, the doctors take the cast off. The wrist is now fixed, and

33

is a strange color and smelly. The pain has also gone. This is how it's supposed to work and, for most of us, it does. It used to for me as well.

Virginia Splat!

The first time my wrist was broken was at a square dance, during a dance called the Virginia Reel. This dance has two rows of men and women, with partners facing each other.

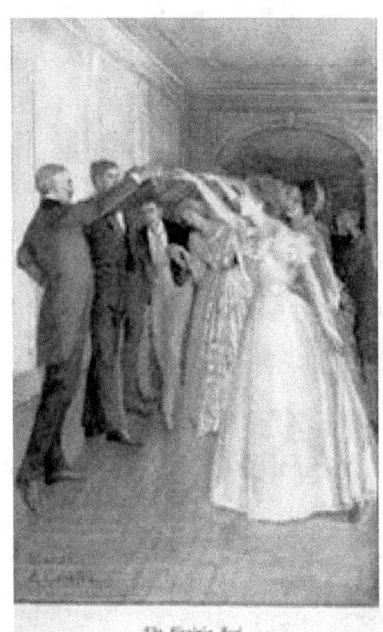

The Virginia Reel.

A part of the dance has a bridge formed by the head couple, the couple closest to the band, and all the other couples go under the raised arms. When it was Ann and my turn, the head man stuck his foot out, tripping me up. The other men, including me, had done this throughout the dance. This time, the head man was a friend and decided to make sure I fell. This is where I use the phrase, with friends like him, who needs an enema? I fell forward with both arms outstretched, and hit the ground with a resounding slap. Even though I hurt, I continued with the dance, because it's not macho to complain. When the dance finished, we drove home and went to bed. By 2am, the pain had ratcheted up to a level I could no longer ignore. I woke Ann and had her take me to the local hospital, where they told me I'd broken the right one and they put a plaster cast on.

The left one they weren't sure about and simply put an ace bandage on. They toyed with the idea of slings on both arms, but couldn't work out how to do so. The wrist followed the normal pattern and, some weeks later, the doctor removed the cast and the wrist was fixed. It was yellow and smelly, but it no longer hurt. For a few minutes, it felt light as I had become used to the extra weight from the cast. After I washed the yellow gunk off, the wrist was back to normal.

Joseph

The memory that sticks with me is from the Sir Andrew Lloyd Webber and Tim Rice musical, Joseph and His Amazing Technicolor Dreamcoat. Ann and I had front row seats and, during the encores, I was on my feet clapping with the rest of the audience. Even through all the lighting, the actors could see the plaster cast on my wrist and kept pointing at me and commenting about my enthusiasm.

I was in pain, but at that moment I was also happy; the memory is one that brings me joy. I don't remember the pain, but do remember the play and the joy of seeing it. I remember the number of encores they got, seven, and the joy of being with Ann. Playing the music CD reminds me of the show, but not the pain. My spirit bubble fills with joy when I hear music from the show. This is how music therapy works. Another line item in my plan of happiness.

The opposite of joy is not pain; I can be in pain and find joy anyway. I can be happy and be hurting. The opposite of joy is unhappiness. A person is sorrowful, miserable, melancholy and gloomy. Someone with constant, chronic pain can also be sorrowful, miserable and gloomy. We can also add depressed, despairing and have lost hope; seeing no light at the end of the tunnel except for a train coming the other way. Filling my spirit bubble with any of these opposites of joy is negatively charging it.

18-year-old girls can be dangerous

The next time I broke my wrist, my recovery didn't follow the expected route, although what happened was humorous in a 'that will teach you' sort of way. It also caused me many reverse joy emotions.

One of my daughter Amy's friends, Amanda, loved to have me tease her and to tease me, even when she was 18. This day, she kept on teasing until she got a response. I eventually jumped from my chair and gave chase. Unfortunately, I managed to slip and everything slowed down.

It was eight months after I'd had major surgery on my left arm. I was aware of the metal plate, three inches down from my shoulder. The doctor had warned me not to damage the arm, as the bone would snap off at the edges of the plate. I was falling to my left and knew how bad that could be. Somehow, I avoided hurting my left arm, but did manage to break my right wrist, the little finger on my left hand and several ribs on both my left and right sides. This accident brought me no joy at all.

It brought joy to Amanda and she mocked me (still does).

You can't splint broken ribs; you simply suffer until they heal. If the pain is too great, you take pain medication. Even without a time machine, I can hear the chorus of sarcastic, snarky comments.

"Oh, what a shame."

"Serves you right!"

"You shouldn't chase 18-year-old girls."

You're right, except years later it still hurts. When this break occurred, I had the devil-spawned disease Reflex Sympathetic Dystrophy (RSD). You may not have heard of this condition, I hadn't and few people I speak to have, either. One reason may be because the medical fraternity doesn't understand the condition.

The original name was Causalgia. You did something and the pain stayed. Science progressed to recognize the Sympathetic Nervous (SNS) and Para Sympathetic Nervous (PNS) systems manage pain.

Simplistically put, one system turns on pain sensors and the other switches them off when everything is ok again. Hence, the sympathetic word, which has nothing to do with anyone having sympathy for you. With RSD, the pain stays.

No one knows why an area affected by RSD hurts as if the trauma recently occurred.

One theory suggests that Norepinephrine, also known as adrenaline, is released from sympathetic nerves and acquires and keeps the capacity to activate and reactivate pain pathways.

Eventually, the RSD sufferer may suffer the trauma pain bilaterally. The pain in the left wrist is now in the right wrist or the right ankle even though that body part has undergone no trauma.

The term RSD, somehow didn't sit right with doctors, possibly because non-doctors can understand it. In the last few years, RSD has become Complex Regional Pain Syndrome (CRPS), a meaningless name. Those of us who suffer, now use the term RSD/CRPS, or stick with the original RSD as I do. It has been with me since 2002, why honor it with a new name?

McGill Pain Index

In 1971 two researchers, Melzack and Torgerson at McGill University in Montreal, Canada developed a scale of rating pain developed. It is a self-report questionnaire that allows individuals to give their doctor a good description of the quality and intensity of pain that they are experiencing. Over the years since, Ronald Melzack and others have developed a pain index chart providing a number for a range of fairly common pain condition. The scores are out of 50 and give some idea how each trauma compares with the others.

Why out of 50? I don't know. It is something I would like to know as well, but I don't have the time to find an answer. The other is what purposeful bone amputation scores. Whatever the maximum number the pain types are out of, it gives a good view of how pain affects each of us. For example, a toothache is considered to be worse than a broken bone. A bruise is worse than both of them, even though this seems counter-intuitive or unlikely. Most of us would probably say it is the other way around. I will trust Melzack, as he has continued to receive recognition and awards for his study and understanding of the mechanisms of pain. He is an expert in psychology due to his studies and explanation of experiencing pain and definitely not any sort of drip under any pressure of any kind.

Sprain	*14*
Arthritis	*18*

Cut	*18*
Bone Fracture	*18*
Toothache	*20*
Shingles	*22*
Bruise	*22*
Phantom limb pain	*24*
Non terminal Cancer	*24*
Chronic back pain	*27*
Fibromyalgia	*29*
Childbirth with training	*35*
Childbirth without training	*37*
Accidental bone amputation	*40*
RSD/CRPS	*45*

RSD is the worst pain there is. I find it unbelievable childbirth scores 35 and RSD 45. Labor scores 10 levels lower? Even accidentally chopping off a finger or a foot, scores as five levels less painful. Not having gone through labor personally, I can't know what mothers suffer as they give birth. I hear they forget until the next time. Having watched Ann through the birth of our three biological children, I know it's no fun! I am also glad that only women go through the "joy of childbirth" otherwise the human race would no longer exist. I don't believe I could deal with the pain even though the chart tells me that RSD is much worse than labor.

I simply cannot see how RSD is 10 levels worse than childbirth, so I asked some women who had both RSD and children. They tell me the notable difference is RSD doesn't stop hurting. Men know a hit in the groin can turn your world black for a few minutes, leaving you writhing. Eventually the groin stops hurting, not RSD.

There are hundreds of symptoms, covering the whole body, reported by RSD sufferers. I intended to add the list here, but it was several pages long and too depressing. I checked yes to over 90% of them. Some symptoms are the opposite of others in the list. This isn't as weird as it may sound, as the disease affects us all differently.

The pain stays

One symptom of my love/hate affair with the disease is that, whenever I've hurt myself since RSD blighted my life, the pain stays forever. Actually, there is no love/hate affair, only a hate/loathe one. Over time, the parts damaged pre-RSD have felt left out and have decided to join in the fun. As you may recall from the list of damaged body parts earlier in this book, I have damaged my body from the top of my head to the bottom of my feet. Every one of these damaged parts hurts as if I just damaged them. If you have ever broken a bone, strained a muscle or cut yourself you may understand and recognize how much pain I am in.

I don't seem to have had a vote in this decision, because I'd have argued against it. But then, who am I to make decisions? Many wives (not mine, of course,) would suggest this isn't a man's role. In the catastrophe caused by Amanda, you could argue a 47-year-old man, chasing an 18-year-old girl got what he deserved. My problem is accepting the fact that the pain stayed. The doctors splinted the wrist, and left the little finger alone and it now sticks out at about a 30 degree angle.

With my broken ribs, they told me to take some pain pills and not to call them in the morning, because there was nothing they could do. I'd have to wait for the ribs to heal by themselves. That night, Ann, Amy and Amanda traveled to a conference, leaving me at home with several little children. That's when the gremlins decided now was the time they needed to pay me a visit in earnest and arrived in groups.

Gremlins

Have you noticed how gremlins wait for the opportunity to make life easier? I expected no problems and had no difficulty with being left with the babies and some broken bones. That is, until bedtime. As soon as I lay down, invisible gremlins jumped on the broken ribs and beat them with red-hot pokers. The pain was unbearable and I sat back up, as quickly as possible.

Sitting or standing caused me no new pain, but the process of lying down was horrible. I hadn't yet learned how to manage pain and so turned into a whimpering little boy. I found and took some of the powerful pain pills, the doctor had prescribed and floated off into La-La land for a while.

Fortunately, the children had been in bed for a couple of hours, so no one missed me. A few weeks passed and the bones knitted, allowing me to lie down without hurting too much. My ribs still hurt now, many years later, but not at the 10/10 level. I am actually happy with that because 10/10 is as bad as it can get.

During this time, my spirit bubble was filled with negative emotions, especially those to do with self-pity and pity parties to which no one came. As I was effectively a single parent of several babies at the time, I had to learn how to release the negative emotions and make my spirit bubble positively charged. This is a positive outcome from being sassed by an 18-year-old girl. The fact the pain is staying is something I need to include in my plan of happiness. I can't ignore it. If I want to positively charge my spirit bubble, I must consider and manage the persistent severe pain, because there is no likelihood of it ever stopping. I have also to deal with the problems caused by the fact that others frequently refuse to accept I have chronic pain.

Pain is subjective and the only way to know how another person feels is with a pain chart. On different days and under different circumstances, for the same part of my body, the pain I suffer ranges from overcast to snow. My goal is to be sunny and joyful, with a positively charged spirit bubble, even when my whole body is at a pain level of 10/10. This can be very hard to do, but that isn't going to stop me keeping on trying.

Pain chart

If I allowed it, the physical pain will fill my spirit bubble with negative emotions, leaving no room for positive emotions. Then there is the spiritual, emotional and mental pain which chronic pain brings.

These wait their turn to jump in quickly when there is space, if I let them. I fight to make myself feel joyful so they can't. To make myself joyful,

	What is your weather today?		
	Sunny	0-1	No pain or only minor annoyance at times
	Partly Cloudy	2-3	Pain beginning to interfere with life but manageable most of the time
	Overcast	4-5	Pain is constant but low intensity
	Showers	6-7	Pain intermittent but interferes with most activities of life. Keeps you entirely from a few activities.
	Sleet	8-9	Many activities difficult due to pain. Sometimes function at lower levels.
	Snow	10	Almost all activity difficult due to pain. You are "snowed in" and most activities are cancelled for the day.

I've learned to begin from where I am and fight back from that place. If I'm snowed in, I have two choices – either stay there forever or try to get out. I can't be melancholy; I can't be gloomy, depressed or unhappy because these all negatively charge my spirit bubble. When this happens the pain quickly becomes a lot worse for me.

I can fight, or I can give in. I choose to not to be a donkey. This is not a reference to a political party, but to the melancholy, miserable and gloomy creature from the A.A. Milne, Winnie-the-Pooh stories.

There are several synonyms for donkey and, other than the ones related to horse, none are positive. They include: - idiot, blockhead, dope, dolt, nitwit, simpleton, numskull, fool, duff, blockhead, knucklehead, nincompoop and lame-brain. Any one of these words defines the person who refuses to fight the problems that prevent them from succeeding.

A wonderful synonym I will use to describe such a person is "zounderkite". This word isn't in use today. Or for a long time. It's a Victorian word for idiot and was used when someone did something unpleasant such as the modern-day habit of cutting us off in traffic.

<u>You</u> have RSD?

Many people, including those with similar pain issues, tell me they're surprised to hear I have RSD, as I seem to be cheerful. What they miss is that finding and displaying joy takes effort, but the choices are to appear cheerful, or show the frightening reality. My plan of happiness says I must be happy.

One problem with RSD is that, how we look on the outside and how it feels on the inside are polar opposites. RSD is a giant iceberg. On the inside, we feel like a soul condemned to hell, while on the outside we look ok.

Regardless of how much I want to scream and shout hysterically, as in the film depictions of lost souls, I choose to do my best, to let joy

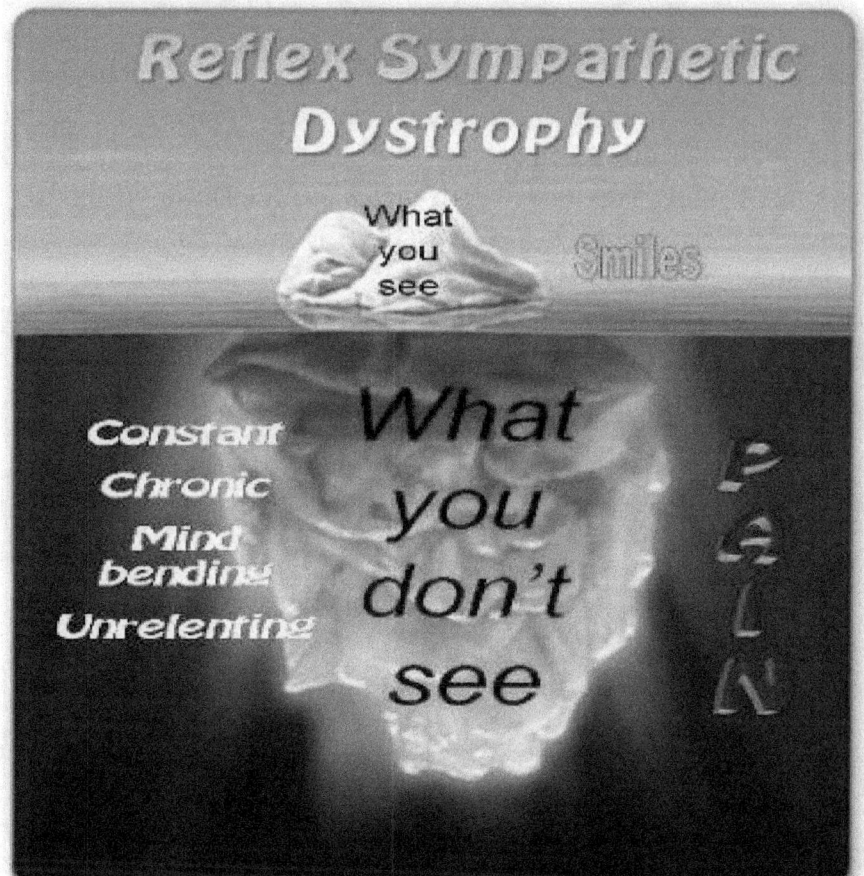

shine through the pain. One way is to not take ownership of the disease. It isn't my RSD, it's the RSD or the <your favorite curse word> RSD.

It doesn't own you! It is the pain I suffer, not **my** pain. I don't want it, I would be more than happy if it went away and I most definitely don't want to claim ownership of it. So it's THE pain and nothing more than that. I don't know or care who owns it, it isn't me! Nor is it you, NOBODY owns pain. We can inflict pain on others, emotional, physical, spiritually or mentally, but nothing we do can actually give us ownership of pain. So why should those of us in pain take ownership of it?

Act as if

The small phrase, "act as if" covers everything talked about in self-help books and programs. The idea is relatively simple. If we want to develop any quality in ourselves, start behaving "as if" we already have that quality. This is a major process in my plan of happiness. If we want to lose weight, *act as if* we have no desire for sweets, bread, pasta and rice. Easy? Of course not! It's as easy as nailing jelly to a tree.

To *act as if,* we use our imagination and pretend or **act as if** what we want to happen is happening, or has happened. In a family situation, this is useful to overcome problems where both spouses may well be in the right, but they can't accept the other person's point of view. If we want our spouse or children to act more loving, respectful, kind or helpful towards you, ask how we'd behave towards them if they were, and act that way. **Act as if** they are, even when they aren't, especially then.

Strange as it may seem or sound, the other person will begin to respond and act in the way we want them to. This isn't an exact science, but it does work when we do it in partnership with the Golden Rule of doing unto others, as we would have them do to us. It works because we give our spirit bubble a powerful positive charge, which can override, or overcome, the other persons negatively charged bubble.

I **act as if** I am not in chronic pain across my whole body. This is hard to do, as my body constantly reminds me that I am. When I am unhappy, I decide to force myself to be happy; to be joyful. I refuse to be miserable and when I fail and am gloomy and miserable I shrug my shoulders. I then force myself out of the funk and refuse to be a zounderkite. I don't worry that I failed; I **act as if** I am happy with the way my life is right now. This is essential when I find that I am, in fact, far from happy with everything that's happening. I need my spirit bubble filled with joy, not negativity, so I will act as if it is. I'm aware this sounds like circular reasoning, but it does work.

Change may take time

Acting **as if** is a psychological trick we can play on others we deal with and it is possible to purposely refuse to change.

If we try it once and once only, then revert back to the "he/she can't change" idea and double down on the negativity, things not only won't improve, they will get worse. It takes time to change and the first time, the other person simply can't believe we're being honest, when we're being nice. They believe it's some sort of ruse to trick them into something. We may have to try dozens of times before we get some movement, some change in their behavior.

We have to keep trying, keep on acting **as if,** because it generally will work. **We** will change and the other person will change. It may take a little time, but it should happen. Even if they don't the changes we have made to ourselves will be sufficient to make a difference so that we will believe things have changed. Even when they haven't **we** will feel so much better.

This is when we might have to decide to lessen our contact with people who have a negatively charged spirit bubble **because** they are draining us of joy and positivity. I suggest we have less contact, for a while, so we can develop a method of (1) positively charging our spirit bubble after being with them and (2) preventing them negatively affecting our spirit bubbles in the future.

Assumptions

Assumptions can be problematical and often cause unhappiness in ourselves and others. We assume we must suffer if we have a broken bone because "everyone" tells us we have a medical condition and will have pain. We may have to endure the pain, but that doesn't mean we have to be unhappy. We can still find joy. We can take medications to manage the pain; we can revel in being taken care of; we can find new hobbies and way to spend our time. We can be joyful anyway, even though the pain is mind-bending.

In March 2002, my family and I were in a car wreck 800 miles from home, in which our 11-year-old daughter Elizabeth died. When we eventually got home, four weeks later, there was a huge outpouring of grief at her school. In fact, every child sent us a letter, even the kids in Kindergarten, telling us how sad they were to hear she was dead. We have several hundred letters, and an expensively bound book the school had made, with the letters from the kids in her class. The school planted a tree in in her memory and had a remembrance service.

On the last day of school, they honored her in the school assembly and had Ann and I attend as guests of honor. Reports of her death were in the school newsletter and the local newspapers. It's inconceivable anyone at Liberty Elementary school wouldn't know Elizabeth was dead, at least that is what I believed. Her friends had all signed her book, so they all knew she had died.

Can I speak to Elizabeth?

During the summer break, a girl called and asked to speak to Elizabeth. My immediate reaction was negative. I asked who was calling and she said she was a friend from school. In as harsh a tone as I could, I said Elizabeth was dead and I didn't appreciate her call.

What I thought we had here was a nasty little girl, getting some perverse pleasure from asking to speak to someone she knew was dead. We could easily build a picture of this nasty little girl, couldn't we? It all depends on the assumptions built into our plan of happiness.

Ann heard the call and asked who it was – I told her and then remembered (we'll call her Suzie) had moved to another state before the spring break holiday when we'd had the accident. She didn't know her friend had died!

Ann called the girl back (her number was on caller id) and spoke with her mother. Suzie was devastated both by the news of Elizabeth's death and by the nasty, heartless and cruel way her daddy had told her. She was also upset I was rude and angry with her, when all she had done was to ask to speak to one of her best friends. Ann explained we'd had several calls from telemarketers recently and I'd assumed this was another one. We sorted out the hurt feelings, talked to Suzie, and tried to help her come to terms with Elizabeth's death.

As with Suzie's phone call, we can appear nasty, not because we are, but because we're trying to deal with our own problems and theirs don't seem that important.

We may believe the other person dislikes us and we're on the defensive because we've heard them say something unpleasant to and about us. We assume this is another example of their unpleasant behavior and now we're acting in a way we believe is justified. They are doing it so I can too. So there! Sounds childish when we put it like that, doesn't it?

Act as if they are doing what we want

The best way, is to assume the other person is NOT being objectionable, not being a zounderkite. Behave **as if** they are nice, regardless of what we think we heard or read, because we **do not** know the back-story. What we may hear or see could make us believe negative things. They're shouting or behaving obnoxiously and are badly behaved. They should, indeed they must, be treated worse than they are behaving. Yes?

An example of knowing how the back-story changed some people's attitude occurred at our sons Andrew's high school graduation. Two little girls became part of our family that day and were misbehaving. Those sitting near us were tutting and giving us evil looks. One woman leaned over, tapped me on the shoulder and demanded I keep my children in check, so she could watch the ceremony. I told her they were foster children, who'd come to live with us a few hours earlier and I had no idea how to calm them down and get them to behave. I'd decided to let them blow off some steam. Most people's attitude changed. Some people still scowled and muttered. I left them to it! These we will call zounderkites

Choose something pleasant

What am I suggesting? If we must make assumptions, choose something pleasant. Choose a positive possibility. Assume the other person is trying to be nice, regardless of what the evidence seems to suggest. Their spirit bubble is filled with unhappiness and negativity, ours doesn't have to be. We may be wrong, but **we** will feel better, because we aren't allowing ourselves to become upset.

It could be that the other person's wife put him in the doghouse, or it's the wife, unhappy over whatever he did. Unless, or until, we know the facts, we can make up whatever happened, so why not choose something that doesn't hurt **our** feelings? After all, we're talking about a plan of happiness. I want my spirit bubble full of positiveness.

I don't mean the problem of cognitive dissonance, where someone is trying to process two contradictory beliefs. Nor am I suggesting pretending something doesn't exist or hasn't happened. We don't know why someone else is being unpleasant to us, so we can choose to make up something positive in relation to ourselves. If I am failing in my goal of keeping my spirit bubble full of joy, there is every possibility I will be a zounderkite and appear miserable and gloomy.

If someone offends us, in person, in print, on the Internet, **act as if** and assume the other person is having a difficult day and they don't want to offend us. Assume they have misspoken, or we have misinterpreted what they said. Ask if we understood them and repeat back what we thought they said, they may apologize and rephrase it.

Having dealt with dozens of children, I know people can be tired, sick or simply out of sorts. They can suck all the positiveness out of other's spirit bubble for miles around, or so it feels. What do we do? We do the hardest task on the planet. We refuse to join in the whine festival and stay sober in all we do. It is hard to stay nice, not shout back, etc. If you've had to deal with tired children, you'll know how hard this can be. Looking for joy, even when there appears to be only pain, requires us to do so and should be part of our plan of happiness.

When others are being unpleasant, **act as if** they have a large peacock feather stuck up their butt and concentrate on that image. This way, we can still fight the pain and find joy. If we are on social media, unfriend them, we don't need that sort of hassle. I do whatever I need to do to is **act as if** I wasn't in pain. I can't make it go away or stop hurting, but acting as if there's no pain, even if I can only manage it for short bursts, is how I get through any day. All that changes is my attitude about its effect on me. I can be upset, or accept it is what it is. I can also be joyful about the image of the other person trying to deal with a peacock feather.

Reality check

We need to expect that **acting as if** requires us to accept things may not change. I know of a number of people who refuse to change even when presented with irrefutable evidence that they're wrong and need to change. Politic activists in today's society aren't the only group of people who probably know they are wrong but don't care. They want the facts to be what they insist they are regardless of how far away from reality that makes them.

Some, what we might consider normal people, won't respond to the **"act as if"** method. When these are family members, we can't use the normal response and stop associating with them. I admit I don't have the answer to this problem.

Most people I have come into contact with have responded to **acting as if**, by changing. The human brain generally prefers not to be in chaos and if it is shown there's a way to overcome and remove the chaos, it will do everything it can to help us change.

Acting <u>as if</u> when others don't change

One area of my life that is hard to deal with using the "**act as if**" method is having RSD. You could assume that, as I am writing a book about fighting pain and finding joy, I already have everything sorted and everyone knows how much I'm suffering and acts accordingly. This unfortunately isn't so. Even those closest to me prefer to **act as if**

I don't have any pain. I am constantly hit on my left arm even though I repeatedly remind others that a soft touch feels like a sledgehammer.

This is one of the toughest parts of finding joy while fighting pain. I have to **act as if** they weren't being cruel and purposefully whacked me. I have to ignore the rolled eyes when I have to find a padded seat instead of sitting on an unpadded one, because of my broken tail bone and IS joint. I have **to act as if** they don't mutter, gripe and complain when I can't pick up my empty dinner plate because my wrist hurts so much. Or carry a gallon container of milk from the car; especially when yesterday I could do so. I have to accept that this may never change and **act as if** it doesn't bother me. In this case, I'm trying to convince myself I'm not upset by the other person's behavior and **act as if** it doesn't bring my immense sorrow. Very hard to do, I know.

What having RSD means to me

To give those without RSD an idea how it feels for those with it, someone wrote a letter to their family in relation *(pun intended)* to the disability. It has appeared in many web sites. The author is unknown and the letter has changed many times. Below is my version of it. I add it here to show what I have to deal with just to exist every day, before I have to try to deal with the problems my wife, 9 children, 9 grandchildren and 3 children-in-law have. I don't want to sound boastful, but theses are my parenting credentials.

This is how I can say we have to act as if others are acting as I want them to, even when it is manifestly obvious to me and anyone else looking, they are not. Regardless of the very real and difficult to deal with things I talk about in this letter, I have no choice but to fight the pain and find joy. It also doesn't mean I shouldn't send this letter and help others realize my spirit bubble really is full of joy, even if they can't see how theirs could be in the same situation.

Dear family member or friend,

I have been diagnosed with RSD, but I'm still a human being. I spend most of my day exhausted and in considerable pain. Sometimes, I don't seem to be much fun to be with, but I'm still me – stuck inside a body no longer working properly. I still worry about my family, my children, my friends, and most of the time – I want to hear you talk about yours, too.

Please understand the difference between "happy" and "healthy". When you have the flu, you probably feel miserable with it. I've been sick for years. I can't be miserable all the time. In fact, I work hard at not being miserable. This means that, if you're talking to me and I sound happy, I'm happy. That's all. It doesn't mean I'm not in a lot of pain, or extremely tired, or I'm getting better. There is also the possibility I am down in the dumps over something other than the pain. Please don't say, "Oh, you're sounding better!" or "But you look so healthy!" I'm coping. I'm making myself sound happy and trying to look normal. If you want to comment on that, please do.

Being able to do something for 10 minutes doesn't mean I can do it for 20 minutes, or an hour.

The fact I managed to do it for 30 minutes yesterday, doesn't mean I can today. With many diseases, either you're paralyzed, or you can move. With RSD, it gets more confusing every day. I don't know how I'll feel when I get up in the morning. Many times, it's from minute to minute.

RSD is variable. One day I can work in the garden, the next day I may have trouble getting to the next room. Please don't attack me by saying, "But you did it before!" or "Oh, come on, I know you can do this!" If you want me to do something, ask if I can. In a similar vein, I may need to cancel an earlier commitment at the last minute. If this happens please don't take it personally. If you can, please try to remember how lucky you are to be physically able to do everything you can do.

Another painful statement I hear a lot is, "You need to push yourself more, try harder..." Sometimes taking part in a single

51

activity, for a short or an extended period can cause more pain than you could ever imagine. Something as simple as putting a ladder up can leave me in agony for hours. You can't always read it on my face, or in my body language.

If I give one of my children or grand-children, a shoulder ride, then pull faces and mutter how much it hurts, it's because it hurts! I'm putting up with the pain for their sake, because they are more important to me than the pain. It doesn't mean I'm feeling better.

I know you find it hard to accept RSD could be 10 levels worse than childbirth, but I didn't come up with the pain level chart, researchers who do not have RSD did.

If you think you have a cure to me, please don't tell me. It isn't because I don't appreciate the thought, and it isn't because I don't want to get well. Lord knows this isn't true. It's likely, if you've heard of it so have I. In some cases, I've been made worse, not better.

This can involve side effects or allergic reactions. It includes failure, which makes me feel worse.

If there were something that cured, or even helped people with RSD, I'd know about it. There is worldwide networking (both on and off the Internet) between people with RSD. If something worked, we'd KNOW. It's not for lack of trying. If, after reading this, you still need to suggest a cure, please do. If it's something new to me, I may discuss it with my doctor. If I seem touchy, it's probably because I am. It isn't how I try to be.

In fact, I try hard to be normal. I hope you'll try to understand. I have been, and am still, going through a lot. If you touch my left arm, no matter how gently, I will jump and pull away from you. I jump and turn away from gentle breezes as well, so please don't take it personally.

RSD is hard to make sense of, unless you have it and even then it makes little sense. It wreaks havoc on the body and the mind. It's exhausting and exasperating. I'm doing my best to cope, and live my life to the best of my ability.

I ask you to bear with me, and accept me as I am. I know it's difficult to understand my situation, but as much as is possible, I'm asking you to try to do so in general. It would make my life a lot easier if you didn't tell me I'm doing nothing, when you feel, if you were me, you'd do more.

Think how you felt the last time you were seriously ill and try to believe me when I tell you, that's every day for me. You got better, I didn't and won't. When you were ill, you didn't want to do anything. Please remember how you felt and accept that I feel no better than you did then. The difference is, this is a good day for me and I don't have too many of them.

I know I'm asking a lot from you, and I thank you for listening. It means a lot to me.

Dave

No comparison

Happiness is contagious... when you reflect happiness, then all others around you catch the happy bug and are happy too.
(Author Jennifer Leese)

Broken ribs and even RSD, pale into insignificance in comparison to the horrors many of our foster children have suffered.

My definition of pain, breaks it into four types. Spiritual, mental, emotional and physical. Spiritual pain occurs when we aren't doing what we believe we should be doing. We think we are an awful parent or child. We know we shouldn't be stealing from our employer, yet we keep on doing so.

I define mental pain as the type of pain treated by medication, such as depression, either short term or long term. This can be caused my physical imbalances in the brain as well.

Emotional pain comes from abuse, either caused by ourselves or others. The death of a loved one is a big emotional pain causing trauma. Another is being the victim of verbal or digital bullying. We can also cause this pain ourselves by having unreasonable expectations of ourselves or others. It can come from other people thinking and saying horrible, viscous things that you believe are untrue. This hurts even more when it is said by those closest to us, who don't believe we suffer pain as much as we do.

Physical pain comes from doing something like breaking a bone or stubbing a toe. We have all suffered some type of physical pain, even if it has only been using a shin to find something in the dark.

Spiritual pain tends to come from us doing things we know we should not be doing; or from not doing things we know we should. This is not the same as OCD – Obsessive Compulsive Disorder. It is more to do with our concept of right and wrong and doing something

54

we know we should not but do it anyway or don't do something we know we should. Spiritual pain is also caused when we are on the receiving end of someone inflicting us with this type of pain. We tend to call spiritual pain guilt and we are all past experts on using the guilt card against others and also on ourselves.

It is possible to be suffering all four types of pain at the same time. I manage to do it many times as I negotiate each day. Because of this, I can help others. I can relate to some of what's happening to them and have empathy. I don't know exactly how they feel, but I have gone through a similarly horrible trauma.

Foster children go through all four as well. As well as any physical pain inflicted by their parents, they may have suffered from emotional pain from what their parents did to them, themselves and others. They wonder what they did and feel guilty for whatever it was. In my experience, the foster parents have no idea what really happened in the child's family. We are just asked if we will take a child. They give us a few details about the child and none about the child's family This means we have little or no idea how to help when they first arrive. We treated them as normal children unless their behavior suggested otherwise. Coming to live with us was a huge emotional and spiritual change for them. They didn't know us and we didn't know them. Sounds like a recipe for disaster, I know. Definitely, life changing.

Two-year-old Raymond's life changed forever when his mother's boyfriend decided to punish Raymond by holding his hand under a running hot tap. He held it there for twenty minutes, until all the skin sloughed off. This excuse for a man, no not a man – he is a male because his genetics say he is. No man would think his punishment was acceptable.

The hand trauma was only part of the agony Raymond suffered. Part of the life-changing event, his mother's boyfriend's horribly unpleasant choices and actions caused that night. One life-changing event the boyfriend doubtless didn't expect was the visit from the police. He was handcuffed and taken to the local jail. His choices and the natural consequence of them, have him convicted as a child abuser.

Raymond also got a trip in a car he was unsure about. This was from the hospital, where his mother took him for treatment of the third degree burns on his hand, to our house, with a social worker.

Our lives also changed with his arrival. We already had several foster children in our home and, whilst the addition of one more normally wouldn't have caused wholesale disruption, Raymond's needs were much more than those of a normal foster child.

To stop the infection spreading, his hand needed constant treatment. He amazed us with the way he handled the treatment without complaint, as we wiped and generally cared for his hand. Each touch was agonizing, yet he hardly ever complained. He'd learned from his mother and her boyfriend that to do so, would cause him more pain. Many of these "people" will beat any child who complains or cries. They only stop when the child is no longer complaining or crying. They quickly learn not to complain in these situations. I say "people" because calling them animals isn't fair to animals.

We had to change the dressings every day and skin would come off with the bandage. It must have hurt horribly, yet all Raymond did was whimper. In the past few years, I've had many surgical procedures, including having needles stuck in the front of my neck, all the way to the spine. I have had this done both sedated and wide awake. The doctor warned me not to move, or to swallow, otherwise I'd be severely hurt, possibly paralyzed. I was not to speak, or they might slice my vocal chords. I was nowhere near as stoic as Raymond was, although I did keep as still as I possibly could.

Raymond's life changed positively and forever, when his mother lost custody. The courts decided she was an unfit mother, as she could have stopped her boyfriend. She had to make a choice between her son and the boyfriend and chose poorly. Raymond left to live with his father's mother, until his dad returned from his tour of duty abroad. The father's commanding officer gave him a leave of absence to visit Raymond, and a warning to bring no dishonor to the Core.

Remember or forget?

It's horrible how Raymond had to suffer such pain and suffering. Fortunately, the outcome was stability, love, and the knowledge he'd no longer have to deal with his mother or her boyfriend. I'm hopeful his spirit bubble has stayed positively charged and he cannot remember much, if anything, about the incident. This hope is unfortunately not founded in fact. I know from personal experience and my 130+ children that we do remember.

Our brains don't move short-term memories to long-term memory storage, until we are about 3-years-old. However, memories of unpleasant experiences **are** stored somewhere in our brains. One of our babies, who was 18-months-old, remembered the horror of what had occurred to her 16 months earlier and she had a breakdown directly related to her memories what happened when she was only two months old. Fortunately for her, we understood what was happening and quickly intervened and managed to calm her down.

Surely not again?

Life can throw problems at you out of the blue or, in the case of my wife Ann, out of a drawer. She found a fishhook in our, then 13-year-old son, Matthew's drawer. It got a good hold and we couldn't get it out. We finished off at the emergency room to have it removed, under a local anesthetic. She suffered no lasting pain, but it's weird how, without warning we can find ourselves with a fishhook stuck in our hand, or something figuratively similar.

I broke my wrist again, doing a mundane task I'd done many times before and since. You'd think I'd have learned my lesson! Less than two years after breaking my wrist the second time, when the same gremlins wanted to inflict more pain on someone's wrist, I bravely volunteered to make sure that no one would ever have to suffer what I have been through.

How different can you get?

This time didn't involve me chasing a beautiful 18-year-old girl, or dancing a square dance. It involved raw sewerage. I believe in keeping my life interesting and how much more different can you get than a square dance, a beautiful girl and raw sewerage? I know we can link a beautiful girl and square dancing, but sewage?

We lived in Texas at the time and two of our older children were at college. Amy at Brigham Young University (BYU) in Provo, Utah and Andrew at BYU in Rexburg, Idaho. After several years in Dallas, we'd forgotten what a winter was like. Dallas only has three seasons, spring, summer and fall. The joke about Rexburg, Idaho is that winter ends on July 1 and begins again after the Independence Day celebrations, 3 days later. When it gets above freezing, the students at BYU Idaho consider it a shorts and tee shirt day. The school colors are blue and white and the student's skin match.

Ann and I decided to visit Andrew and Amy in February 2005. We packed our camper and began the 1500-mile trip to Utah and Idaho in 80-degree weather.

In Rexburg, our third night there, the temperature dropped down to 8f (-13C). The propane tank was empty and the camper water and sewer tanks were solid blocks of ice. We couldn't use the on-board bathroom, a major benefit of an RV when children are along for the trip. It's essential, when you park outside a University dorm with no public bathrooms within walking distance. This lack is an impossible inconvenience for our two sons and me. For Ann and my daughter it was insurmountable.

That hurt

We had no choice but to leave and head towards Provo, with a seriously frozen camper, leaving a disappointed Andrew behind. He'd expected us to stay at least another night.

In Idaho Falls, we pulled into a Kamp of America to have another go at freeing the valves. I squatted in the middle of the dump station which has a one brick high wall around the sewer trap. The gray tank, with water from the sinks and shower refused to budge, so I moved to the black water tank, with the sewage.

This valve moved a little and I pulled harder. I'm on my haunches, with one hand on either side of the release valve, exerting all my puny strength. Something had to give. The ice refused to yield. I wasn't stopping. The handle thought, "This is too much for me to handle!" and both sides snapped off. I fell backwards, hitting my right wrist on the barrier bricks.

There was an audible crack and I knew I'd broken the wrist. I dropped the bits of handle on the ground in disgust. I got up, managed to shut the door over the valves and climb back into the cab of the camper. My wrist hurt horribly and the hand was totally limp and wobbly. We found a gas station selling propane and asked for directions to the local hospital.

My hand and arm were X-rayed and there we go, another cast! The doctor told me the bricks had snapped the wrist clean off the arm bones and was the worst he'd ever seen. I enjoy succeeding, but am irritated I can do so well at this. This ability is not part of my plan of happiness, but I must deal with it too often. My trip to the hospital meant we couldn't drive to Provo that night. Andrew got his wish and we stayed another night with him. I have no idea where, as I was drugged up with pain medications.

The snow melted.

The next morning, we headed south to visit Amy in Provo, Utah. The two campuses are approximately 310 miles apart, through some impressive mountain ranges. The cast and sling meant I could no longer drive, so Ann had to drive the 310 miles. She had no difficulty, which was good, because the doctor had prescribed Dilaudid for the pain. This is a morphine derivative, which gets rid of the pain and most of your ability to think.

As we headed south, 5F became 35F. Once at the KOA in Provo, I hooked the camper to the sewerage, water and electricity. I wondered how I'd open the valves, with only one working hand when I'd failed so epically with two.

I was surprised when a pair of pliers easily opened the black water valve. I was amazed and confused when nothing came out. I checked the tank levels in the camper and it showed empty. The obvious tap on the dials still showed empty. The gray water tank showed full, but not the black one. Outside, I pulled the gray water valve open and the water rushed out. The black tank had been full the day before. I must have opened the valve a little in Idaho Falls. As it had got warmer, the tank's contents had melted and leaked out the slightly opened valve. I laughed as I thought about what must have happened. I will never know if anyone recognized what was coming their way, but the thought of it makes me want to laugh now, even though I wouldn't have, if I had been on the receiving end.

What is she throwing at us?

The warmer weather had turned all the snow on the road to slush. Ann emptied the camper's windshield washer reservoir, clearing the slush and crud thrown up by other vehicles. Those behind us had slush, crud and sewerage thrown at them. A truly gross and unpleasant thought. Had they known what we were throwing at them, they'd have been right to call us zounderkites.

It shows how we can find joy in the strangest of places and situations. The joy from the silliness of what had happened overwhelmed the "oh poor me" feeling. My left arm already hurt and now my right wrist was in a cast. I wanted to drive some journey home, but Ann didn't want me to take the risk, so I sat in the passenger seat and visited La-la land.

I now had two useless arms and being zoned out prevented me from thinking too much about that unpleasant situation. The next few months in a cast were itchy and I waited for the pain to stop. I'm still waiting. The pain does subside from time to time, but it also ramps up so high that I can't even lift a dinner plate, without so much pain I have to give up and ask someone to help. The doctors tell me not to lift more than 10 pounds with either hand.

Victims

Happiness is when what you think, what you say, and what you do are in harmony. (Mahatma Gandhi.)

I'm often told to stop being a victim. Most people are referring to the car accident my family had in March 2002. People tell me RSD is all in the head and has nothing to do with vasoconstriction the SNS and PNS cause around the trauma site. Apparently, the pain is caused by thinking about the accident.

It would be spectacular, fantastic, brilliant and amazing if they were correct, and, with the right positive mental attitude, all the pain magically vanished. Devastatingly, it can't, because the pain is real, even though others believe it should be gone, because the bandages, casts, etc. have gone. Most of us are unsympathetic towards those who say their central, sympathetic and parasympathetic nervous systems are out of whack, although having my system in whack doesn't sound much better.

Positive Mental Attitude

A positive mental attitude (PMA) **is** useful however, when managing pain. If we want it to go down, we must **want** the pain to go down. With chronic pain it doesn't go away, we must accept the situation and work out how to handle everything.

Positiveness will positively charge our spirit bubbles, but we must also be sensible and reasonable. Many conditions are invisible and the only way anyone knows we're unwell is because we tell them. When someone has appendicitis, they have this same issue. A surgeon can cut us open, remove the appendix and stitch you back up. Only then can they 100% confirm the appendix was the problem. Once the surgery pain goes away, the patient is OK.

No matter how positive we are, we can't ignore appendicitis, unless a slow painful death is in our plan if happiness. A positive attitude will **not** make the pain go away. Only a skilled surgeon and his sharp knife can do that. Ignore the pain, and we'll die horribly.

Another example, one I know of personally, is kidney stones. There's no external evidence, only the sufferer writhing in agony. I'd had RSD for several years, when I first suffered with a kidney stone and was unpleasantly surprised at how much it hurt. A kidney stone is treated with powerful pain medication, until it passes out the urethra, at which point the pain stops, it literally has passed. They gave me a sieve to pee through, so I could catch the stone. When the pain doesn't stop and you've exhausted all medical possibilities, we must rethink how we do everything, and how it will affect your pain levels. It's a full-time job, with no vacations, terrible benefits, and no way to quit.

Even though it may sound as if I'm complaining and saying, "Oh poor me!" it does **not** make me a victim. A victim purposefully keeps their spirit bubble full of unhappiness and negativity.

Victim

Let's return to my computer and look up the word victim in an on-line dictionary. As both of my wrists hurt constantly, I'm grateful we no longer use heavy dictionaries, because I'd have to complain.

1. A person who has been attacked, injured, robbed, or killed by someone else.
2. A person who is cheated or fooled by someone else.
3. Someone or something harmed by an unpleasant event (such as an illness or accident)

I'm not dead, I've not been attacked; I've been robbed a couple of times and I've been cheated and fooled by someone else. I've been hurt in accidents many times and they all still hurt, so I must be a victim. Yes?

In the media, in books, and on the Internet, you'll find many articles on victim mentality. Most define it as a condition where the pain is mental, not physical. A person with a victim mentality may automatically blame everything on someone else and take no personal responsibility. They carry their victim emotional baggage everywhere.

Victim mentality = stuck!

Victim mentality occurs when people can't move on from a trauma and become angry at the situations in which they find themselves. If your friend calls and says she can't go out with you, you believe she's always canceling. You don't, or won't, see how you calling her at the last minute and leaving a message means she honestly can't go with you.

Life can seem easier using the blame game, but it isn't. If we're sick, we blame the other person. Everything's the other person's fault. The problem is, blaming others moves us backwards and we become locked in a cycle, where we blame someone else for that too. Often, others have no idea they've hurt us. In some cases, they'd apologize and put everything right. Even when they do, though, the "stuck" victim will want to stay with the blame game.

The trauma happened in the past. Blaming others or ourselves needs to be left there. If not, we're stuck being a victim of something that can't un-happen.

Does this condition exist?

Does this mental condition exist? Unfortunately, for those who've suffered trauma, yes, and not merely because the experts say so. I've been there and have the t-shirt. I've put weight on, so the t-shirt no longer fits. Those with the condition have negatively charged spirit bubbles and unless they work to change to it, they will stay victims.

I've learned to accept what happened and get on with my life, even with the physical pain, all day, every day, often 10/10 over my whole body. Remember, the experts tell me to expect the RSD to get worse. Except, an ex is a has been and a spurt is a drip under pressure. I'm not a victim I'm a survivor. My plan of happiness has clauses and processes to make sure I know this. Just because the experts are correct and the RSD has spread and is worse doesn't mean I have to wait around for it to happen. Ok, it will get worse, I'll deal with it, if and when that happens, I'm not about to sink into a pit of misery because in 5 years time I'll hurt more than I currently do. What will that achieve? Nothing! Absolutely nothing!

Retelling our story

Other experts claim talking about our ordeals automatically means we're a victim, because we want pity. They claim we tell and retell the story, because the issues are now part of our identity. My response is "go be a drip under pressure somewhere else". It's part of my past but most definitely not part of my identity. It does **not** define me! I repeat stories where I finished off breaking bones or otherwise hurting myself not so I can ruminate on them, but because I enjoy telling them and always bring out the humorous parts of the story. I believe I can help others in pain. A small warning, if I spend an excessive amount time thinking about the trauma, I can slip into victim mode and then the pain levels increase.

I've been to many faith promoting, uplifting meetings, where the speaker has been to the gates of hell and lived to tell the tale. They tell people how they recovered and can now get on with their lives, as if the trauma had never happened. They aren't victims; they're survivors and are sharing what they did to become one, because they want to help others survive. Their plan of happiness is fulfilled, when they share their journey and their solutions.

The speaker may have suffered as much as Job, and clawed their way back. Badly injured people have overcome mountainous obstacles, to be able to live a full life with prosthetic arms and legs, often totally different from the one they lived before. Each has had to overcome the trauma and the mental, emotional and spiritual blame game that occurs afterwards. They acknowledge what life has done to them and have decided to get on with their lives. They aren't victims.

None of these truly wonderful, uplifting stories fully helps me. The speakers are to be applauded for their efforts, but my situation is different. I'm trying to handle real and constant pain and despite this, find joy in all aspects of life anyway. I'm not a sufferer of victim mentality; I'm the victim of a painful condition, a survivor who must find a way to be joyful, even when in pain.

The paraplegic and quadriplegic people are missing limbs or the use of them. My issues are invisible, but as real and painful. I do find it somewhat odd that some people will try to link and compare conditions. It is a fact of life that a paraplegic is suffering something different from what I am dealing with. However, their being in pain has no effect on how much pain I am suffering. The same is true for them. Suggesting that I will somehow feel better about the holes in my shoes when I look at the man with no shoes. This simply does not work, it is the Brussels Sprouts argument again. The person in Africa will be no more or less hungry if I eat my Brussels Sprouts because if I don't eat them, they will be thrown away, not sent to the hungry person.

If handled correctly what it could do is help to change our attitude and see how lucky we are to have sufficient to eat and at least try the vegetable. Being forced to eat Brussels Sprouts fills our spirit bubble with negativity and unhappiness. As an adult we need to find a way to recharge our bubbles and face Brussels Sprouts so they make us happy.

Living in the now

The trick to finding joy in pain, is to carry on, regardless of what others say or think, and to live in the now. This is the only way to overcome what has occurred because, unless you have a time machine, the past isn't accessible. We can no more change a past event, than you can make me write your name here. There's no rewind button; nor a fast-forward button. Now is all there is and joy comes from doing our best, right now. We can't wait for tomorrow either.

We can change the present and shape the future. Yet, even though living in the now isn't optional, many of us try to live in the past. Today may well be the 5,293rd day in a row that morning has begun with tiredness and pain, but we will make the most of it. Tomorrow it will probably be day 5,294th day with tiredness and pain, so we may as well just do everything we can to enjoy today.

Change the words

Living in the moment, involves a new vocabulary, using softer words. The statements sound and look similar, but the new phrases are positive and move away from victim-hood. I have them written in my plan of happiness to remind me daily.

- **Dislike** instead of *hate*.
- **Discomfort** instead of *pain*.
- **Remember to**, instead of *don't forget*.
- *I'll try*, becomes **I can**.
- *Never give up*, becomes **keep on going**.
- *It is what it is* turns into **it is what I choose it to be**.
- **I am courageous**, instead of I *can face my fear*.
- *Don't worry* becomes **focus on a solution**
- *What can I do?* Becomes **I can do this**.

The words have the same meaning but the bold ones are positive.

With RSD, victim-hood is easy to achieve, especially with medicating to the level the pain goes away. Unfortunately, we're permanently in La-la land and don't have a life. I tried it, but didn't enjoy being permanently zoned out and chose to find a balance, where I am still in pain but it's manageable, and my brain still works.

We must choose to find that balance and take an unpleasant situation and, either turn into something we do like, or find a way to manage it. This may mean acting as if the unpleasant things people are doing or saying to us doesn't bother us.

66

Our spirit bubble needs to stay filled with joy if we ever want to succeed at fighting the pain. This is especially so when everything and everyone doesn't just seem to be fighting against you, they actually are sucking out the joy and filling your spirit bubble with negativity. I can testify how hard that can be, but it is essential we treat the non physical pain in the same way as the physical pain and somehow fill our spirit bubble back up again with as much joy as we possibly can.

Roles and Responsibilities

In such a home, parents are loved and not dreaded; they are appreciated and not feared. And children are regarded as gifts of the Lord, to be cared for, nurtured, encouraged, and directed.
Gordon B. Hinckley

My plan of happiness has a list of roles and responsibilities I play, or have played. As a family member, I play several roles,.

At 10, I played the following roles: - Son, Brother, Grandson, Nephew.

At 20, we could add fiance.

At 30, we remove fiance and add husband, son-in-law, and father.

At 60, I play the following: - Husband, Father, Brother, Uncle, Brother-in-law, Father-in-law, Grandfather, GrandUncle.

As I only had one Aunt and Uncle and they had no children, I haven't played the role of Cousin. If I go back a generation I could include the roles of half cousins etc.

I'm no longer a Son-in-law, Grandson or Nephew.

In our social lives, the roles we play depend on what we are doing. If we play sports, the position we play decides the role we have.

Our role may be as a friend or confidant. There are some people with whom we are close friends, others who are only acquaintances and yet others who are friends of friends. The way in which we behave with each of these groups and the roles we play can vary enormously.

As a dog owner, I have roles regarding their behavior. I may not want to have dogs, but Ann and the children do and therefore must accept the roles.

Roles and responsibilities at work

At 18, I was a new employee at a bank.

At 26, I was a Data Processing manager with several staff and a department to manage.

At 30, I had my own company with responsibility for my staff and the day-to-day running of a company. I also had responsibilities towards my customers and suppliers.

At 40, I was a consultant responsible only for myself but responding to the companies for whom I consulted.

At 60, I'm retired.

I've no idea where I'll be in 20 years time.

In the community

Our biggest roles in the community are as voter and taxpayer. Even if we are unemployed, we still pay taxes. Other roles we can play in the community depend on the level of our involvement. We may be a school governor, a local politician, or even a national politician. We may be on the local neighborhood watch committee. If we attend church, we may be a leader or a Sunday School teacher, as well as a member of the congregation, which itself is a role.

Multiple roles

There's some measure of overlap in each area; we can define ourselves as playing roles in each of them – sometimes several at the same time. For example, at a family reunion, we may be son, father, grandson, nephew, brother-in-law and host all at the same time. Depending on who we're talking to, or dealing with, we may well behave differently in what are the same situations. Once, I was husband, father, son-in-law and grandfather all at the same time. When someone said "Dad" any one of four of us could respond; me, my father-in-law or either of my sons. Granddad could be my father-in-law or me. The only role with one person was great granddad. My father-in-law was fulfilling this role, along with granddad, father and father-in-law. This multi-role situation is common.

Responsibilities

Along with the roles we play are responsibilities or obligations.

As a husband and father, I'm responsible for providing a home, money for food, to pay the bills, etc.

As a member of society, I have the responsibility to obey the laws of the land, such as driving at or below to the speed limit, or pay taxes.

The roles and responsibilities stored in our plan of happiness help us make decisions. For example, if a family member asks me for help, I may make a different decision depending on who it is. If an old relative asked for my help with her shopping, I'm more likely to agree than I would if it was my fully fit younger brother. I decide to pay taxes because I'm a responsible citizen. I also choose to do so because it's dangerous not to, I could go to jail if I don't pay them.

Which set of roles and responsibilities are the most important? That it is a purely personal question, I think. My personal top two roles, the ones most important to me are husband and father.

Is fatherhood disposable?

In today's crazy world it appears to be acceptable to argue I am completely wrong thinking this. We live in a throwaway world where everything is disposable. Fast food is not the only example, but it's a good one we can all relate to. Mobile phones are another. We buy a phone knowing we'll be getting rid of it within a year, possibly two. If our car can be changed when it becomes banged up and rusty, why can't we change out our relationships in the same way? When we suffer pain from it, shouldn't we simply ignore we ever had the relationship?

If our spouse has aged and is no longer as appealing as they were when we first met them, why not change them for a newer better looking model? If our children become too much of a problem, why should we bother continuing with them? Everything is disposable, why not this? It is a common occurrence in today's society, both men and women leaping out of their marriage for a younger person, regardless of how many other people, including their children, are hurt.

You may disagree with me about how long we have to play the role of a father. Some people claim it ends when the child is legally an adult. Their idea is that an adult is capable of looking after themselves, so why should I have to help my offspring who are now adults? I suffer from constant, chronic pain why should I?

I know of some parents who, in my opinion, do not deserve the title. This is because they evicted their children from the family home as an 18th birthday present. What an entrance to the adult world! Foster children automatically find this happening when they reach 18 and have not been adopted. The state takes the attitude that 18-year-olds are adults and they can look after themselves. Same attitude.

One family gave a few weeks warning, others have given no warning. One child showed up at our front door with her bags and in tears. It would seem to me that these non-parents decided many years ago that the hassles their children gave them as teenagers was only temporary, because it would end at their 18th birthday. At least they didn't have to plan any 18th birthday celebrations. Both the parents and the children spirit bubbles must have been full of negativeness.

What is a father?

The third Sunday in June is Father's Day and the day we get to tell our fathers how grateful we are for them. Obviously, how grateful we are depends on how well our father behaved towards us. Do we think they are worthy of our appreciation? How good a father have they been? I believe that the fathers planning to evict their children on the child's 18th birthday definitely don't deserve appreciation.

A real father, a real man would never do this.

I cannot speak for you as I don't know you and your situation, but I hope your children never have a problem picking a Father's Day card, or a Mother's Day card, because the sentiment on and in the card is totally false. I know of people who have this problem every year, they could never sign their name to something that has never been true. They want to, but their father was never a real man. He was a male. Their mother was a female, not a woman.

According to the media, men are bumbling fools who have no idea how to change a diaper, or look after children in any way. He is, at best, an idiot obsessed with sports and women's bodies, not necessarily his wife's. According to Hollywood and television shows, he is of no real use to anyone, except as the person who supplied the seed.

I totally disagree. Fatherhood is the opposite of what society says. I think a father is a real man, worthy of the title "dad", someone who gives all he has to his children expecting nothing in exchange but love.

One of my daughters recently got the news that no one likes to hear, her best friend was moving. My immediate responsibility was to cuddle her. This was a problem because both arms hurt severely and cuddling her, hurt me quite a bit. I did what any good dad would do, I ignored the pain. My needs and my wants were overridden by her needs at that moment. She is important to me and giving up my time and accepting the pain will increase for a while are worth doing.

Not just a seed distributor

A Father is not just the person who supplied the seed and a Mother is not just the person who supplied the egg and the growing space. I believe there's a lot more than that in the role of being a parent. To repeat myself, a father is someone who gives all he has to his children, expecting nothing in exchange but love. The same is true of a mom. The only difference I can see is that a mother is someone who gives all she has to her children, also expecting nothing in exchange but love and, occasionally, hugs and chocolate. Given the choice many mothers may argue that given the choice they'd have the chocolates. My experience tells me otherwise.

Then there's pain

To go with each of my roles and responsibilities I also have constant chronic pain. I have to balance everything, because I'm limited in my ability to do most of it. I can't ignore things because there's a lot I must do.

Not being able to do what I want causes me emotional and spiritual pain and fills my spirit bubble with negative emotions. I don't want this, so I accept I can't do everything and concentrate on what is most important and what is possible and do that. Not only concentrate on them, celebrate I can. It's like the problem I have with dogs. I don't want to be a dog owner, yet I have three. I work around the problem and make it work. I don't want to be melancholy about it; nor do I want to be unhappy.

The dog went off

Some of our foster children have also had problems with dogs. When they come to live with us, life is very different; they have to adjust to new people, odd accents, often different skin color, etc. etc. Serenity and Juan had to adjust to a house with four other children and our Australian Shepherd, Misty, a big dog with a loud bark and a direct connection to the front door. We knew when someone was at the front door, because the dog went off. This can be useful when we're in the basement and don't hear the doorbell. It's irritating when the dog goes off because she sees a neighbor's dog, or is surprised to see the buffalo which have been in our neighbors' yard since we moved into the house and I've no idea why she's surprised to see them. I often wonder if she's barking at something in China, because she starts barking, yet there's no one at the door, no one in the street, no neighborhood dogs invading her domain and no buffalo visible and she wasn't trying to steal my seat. She had to be barking at someone or something. I couldn't see anything yet she kept on doing it.

Misty's barking made Juan's life difficult and he had a problem each time she went off. He'd give a good impression of Tom, of Tom and Jerry fame, jumping out of his skin, then running as fast as he could up the stairs. If Misty were blocking his way, he'd scream. The dog would look at him with a bemused look that asked, "What's your problem?" and back off. She'd lived through some 90 foster children

73

and none had ever behaved as oddly. Being upstairs, didn't resolve Juan's problems; he had to come back down again. He'd look around and, if the dog was there, he screamed. The dog was usually there and so, each morning was a problem. He'd run, screaming up and down the stairs, even when the dog was at the other end of the house. Fortunately, he never thought of getting to the basement and trying to run screaming up and down those stairs as well.

Foster Dog

If a dog could be involved in fostering, Misty has played the role wonderfully well. She's allowed them to use her as a pillow, a punch bag, a teddy bear, a step stool, a rocking horse, a swimming partner and general dog's body. If she could talk, Misty would tell you she plays the role of Defender in Chief as well. She's never complained about anything a child does. The most she's done is whine when, whatever they were doing to her, hurt too much.

When Juan lived with us, she taught him not to fear her. This was useful, because the family who adopted him had a dog and he was now used to one. We helped Juan to live in the now and learn to deal with Misty, a dog with a mission to make children's life joyful. She succeeded so well, Juan no longer felt scared of dogs. Dogs no longer filled his spirit bubble with fear, anxiety and trepidation. They now filled it with happiness and pleasure. With Misty's help, he rewrote his plan of happiness and now looks at dogs through different eyes.

Empathy

The benefit, if that could ever be the right word from having anything unpleasant occur, is that once **we've** learned to handle and manage the trauma, we can help others in similar situations. We can't completely understand how they feel. What we can do, though, is have empathy. Empathy is understanding someone else's condition, from his or her perspective, not ours. We place ourselves in their shoes and imagine what they're experiencing. It's asking, *"What's it like to be them, right now?"* not *"Why are they like this?"* or *"what makes them do that?"* It's even different from compassion and sympathy.

We may know how we felt, when we suffered through a similar episode, and can recognize how they must feel. Even then, we can help the most by being a listening ear. Someone who is willing to let them talk without interruption.

Empathy is the most advanced of all communication skills, the least understood and the hardest to master. It's trying to understand and accept another person's feelings, needs and concerns, even when we may not have suffered anything remotely similar. Or even when we have done so.

I've learned that I know nothing beyond what happened to me. We **cannot know** what is happening in someone else's lives. Even those closest to us don't experience the same event the same way we do. They may even come to different conclusions over what occurred. This happened in the horrible car wreck my family was involved in 2002. It was different for us all, even though it was the same event happening to us all at the same time, in the same place. I even tell a different story about it, depending on who I'm talking to. The story is the same, I just tell certain parts of the story and this possibly makes it sound different to somebody who only ever hears that part of the story.

Find something positive

Whatever the problem may be, finding something positive, a figurative light at the end of the tunnel, can help us find joy even when we're in pain. Regardless of whether the pain is physical, mental, spiritual or emotional. This is how I can help others. I may not know exactly how something affected and is still affecting someone else, but I do know how the same or a similar experience affected me and how I managed to find joy. This is where I can be empathetic.

A while ago, some neighbors suffered the indignity of being evicted from their house. Their children tried to help and held a garage sale to raise enough money to pay the debt. They unfortunately couldn't do so.

We don't know what led to the sheriff and the constables showing up, sticking 'Do Not Trespass' notices on the house doors, and

75

threatening jail to anyone entering the property without permission. We know what people told us, but only our ex-neighbors know exactly what happened. What we could do is be empathetic and tell them how sorry we were over what was happening to them. We could help them remove their furniture etc, etc.

Empathy is helping others fight pain and find joy.

Empathy is not being interested in how someone screwed up so badly, or how much they deserve to suffer. Empathy is helping others find joy in pain, regardless of how they finished off there. The situation they are now in is where they need to find joy. Even when the pain **may** be the result of something they could have done to prevent it, like paying the mortgage.

Unless you have a permanent, constant, untreatable, chronic condition, the pain will eventually go away. Even though I have RSD, my plan of happiness states I will have empathy for others wherever, however and whenever I can.

We all need to find joy even when our circumstances are horrible. We start from where we find ourselves each morning and find joy anyway. We don't compare, because where **we** are, is where **we** start. This is where we're unique. No one else is starting from where we are.

If we're trying to help a person in pain, we need to remember **they** are the one in pain, **not us**. Their roles and responsibilities are different from ours. The road they're traveling is different from the one we're on. The circumstances leading to our paths crossing are unique to us.

When we need to give empathy, the other person's spirit bubble is negatively charged. It is therefore essential ours stays positively charged. If not, their negativity could overwhelm us and any advice we give, may be tinged with anger, or some other negative emotion.

Empathy is trying to give service to someone who is hurting from trauma happening to **them.** Using the opportunity to talk about our problems or to suggest they are somehow wrong feeling how they do, could quickly make thing worse for them or us. As this cannot be our plan, we should plan what to say and do beforehand.

Being on the wrong end of empathy

Suffering from chronic pain can often mean we are on the wrong end of empathy. Others can't or won't accept that we have any problem and can't or won't be nice to us and often are unpleasant to us. This is where we need to know how empathy is supposed to work, so we can have some hope of understanding things from the other's point of view, even when we are the one suffering. Knowing what the other person is **supposed** to do is helpful in dealing with them when they aren't. Some of us simply don't have the talent.

1. Listen without distraction. If we're playing on our phone or watching the television we're obviously not giving our attention.

2. Try to maintain eye contact. Don't stare because that becomes uncomfortable. If we don't maintain eye contact our gaze may finish off drifting everywhere, proving to the other person we don't really care.

3. Reflection. Rephrasing and repeating back what we believe we heard. This is key because it's very possible we've overlaid our emotions onto what they said and have misunderstood their intent.

4. Open up. If we're honest in our desire to help we need to share our emotions and our credentials. We need to show we've experienced something similar to what we're trying to help the other person with. For example, I personally can't help any of my daughters with the pain associated with giving birth. What I know about labor has all been second hand, so it's possible I may not be too empathetic.

With all other pains including many emotional, mental and spiritual pains I have firsthand, personal experience.

5. Allow the other person time to talk. Don't wait until they pause, so we can tell our story. If we want to help them, we want to be able to put ourselves in their shoes. As only they know how that feels, we need to give them the time to speak.

6. Fill our own spirit bubble with positiveness before we try to help. Their spirit bubble will probably be filled with negative emotions and we'll want to overwhelm these emotions and not be overwhelmed ourselves. Empathy is being able to respond appropriately to the other person's apparent mental state.

7. Use "I statements". This is what I did when I was going through my problem. It worked for me. Have you tried it? This is the purpose of this book; how I am Fighting Pain Finding Joy. If the other person says they have and it didn't work or they aren't interested in trying, don't take it personally. Don't allow their negativity to overwhelm you.

If the other person is not following these steps they don't have empathy for us and we'd be better off stopping trying. They may have other talents but empathy isn't one of them. Expecting them to be able to have some, will help neither of us. They are unlikely to change.

David Alan Gray

Wrong choice of roads

***Happiness is the meaning and the purpose of life, the whole aim
and end of human existence. (Aristotle)***

I can be upset because I didn't choose the road I'm on; I wanted a
different road. I want to be on a different one right now! Unfortunately
for me, no one listens; no one cares; they have their own problems to
deal with. We **must** follow the path we find ourselves on. We can try
to turn around and find another road, but that may not be possible.

I had an experience while on vacation in Moab, Utah proving this
to me. It showed me how to accept what has happened and that at

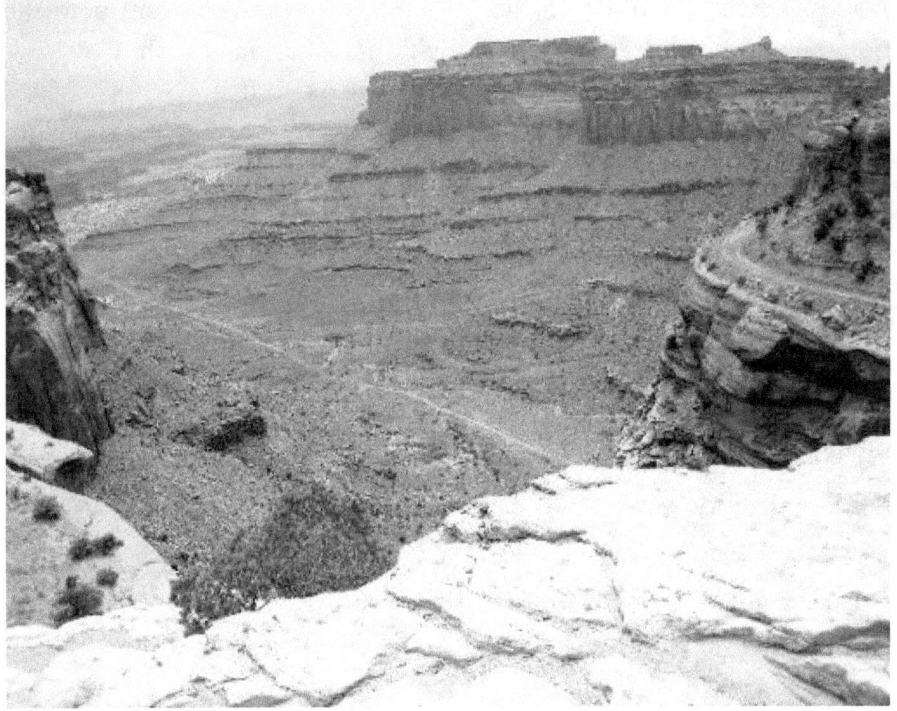

times, there is no turning back. Someone else chose the road we are

79

on; they may have decided without asking our opinion, our input, or even our permission. Nevertheless, we are on this road.

My family was vacationing in southern Utah, where there are several State and National Parks. If you haven't had the chance to go there, I'd recommend you put them on your bucket list.

On a visit to the oddly named Dead Horse Point State Park, we could see a road running across the desert, some 2,000 feet below us. The map showed we could get onto this road from Canyonlands State Park and drive across the desert, to a place called Potash, then to Moab and our hotel. Dead Horse Point State Park has a dramatic overlook of the Colorado River and Canyonlands National Park. This sentence is from the tourist department, not me, but I agree the overlook **is** spectacular. The park's name comes from its use as a natural corral by cowboys, in the 19th century. One legend says cowboys rounded up horses, herded them across the 30 yards wide neck of land onto the point, and fenced off the entrance with branches and brush. Cowboys chose the horses they wanted and let the others go free.

Another legend says they spooked the remaining horses, which all fell off the cliffs. Another suggestion is they were left corralled on the waterless point, where they died of thirst within view of the Colorado River, 2,000 feet below. Whatever the reason for the name, there is a spectacular view.

If you think Dead Horse Point is a weird name for a national park, go look up *Head-Smashed-In Buffalo Jump National Historic Site of Canada*. I'll wait here. We were confident that driving along the road we could see, both on the map and below on the canyon floor, was an excellent idea.

I'll drive

I'd been suffering from RSD for 5 years and was still in pain from a recent fall down some stairs, so Ann was doing most of the driving. For this trip, I decided to ignore the pain and do the driving. Chauvinistic, I know, but Ann didn't want to drive anyway.

We headed for the trail-head in our 4-wheel drive Suburban with our four youngest children. We had no idea what to expect, but assumed a steep, short trip. The road was steep, but from the top, to the valley floor we drove several miles.

The first half-mile was a somewhat level and straight dirt track, some 30 feet wide. This is easy, we thought. Then the road made a 120 degree turn and changed to a narrow potholed one, heading down the side of the mountain at a steep angle. The track was about 18 inches wider than the car, with a 2,000-foot drop to the canyon floor. Having made this first turn, we couldn't turn around, and driving the turn backwards looked far too dangerous. We were committed to the journey down, whether we wanted to or not.

We were on a narrow road with no room for error, and needed to stay on the mountain side of the road. We had to avoid the potholes, all the time staying away from the edge. In several places, there was a five-foot drop on the mountain side and we had to avoid these as well. Falling off the five-foot side could have been a problem, as it may have been next to impossible to get back out. Not as catastrophic, though, as falling off the 2,000-foot side, this doubtless would have been fatal! We'd have created a new name for the park, "Head smashed in Suburban Drop."

Ann and the children on the passenger side had the worst visual part of the journey. All I could see was the road ahead, the cliff walls to my left and, to the right, in the distance, the canyon floor. Ann could see straight down to the canyon floor.

Having made the choice of driving down, we couldn't unmake the decision. We had to continue along the perilous road I'd selected, and hope. At some points, the road was relatively flat and easy, but would quickly change back to steep, narrow and full of potholes. Once down, we followed the desert road, until we came to a junction, where someone had put up a signpost pointing to Potash and Moab. Without the sign, we may have become lost in the desert. This was the last guidepost we saw. After that, we had to guess where the roadway was.

All we had as a guide were tire tracks. Many times, we took the wrong "road", finishing off on dry riverbeds. A few times, we had to negotiate some large inclines across stretches of rock. Fortunately, the car has a high clearance and there were no drops greater than 3 feet. At one point, we were at the bottom of a dam made from concrete, some 40 feet wide and 100 feet high. I didn't wait around to find out how much water may be around. We returned to the point there had been three pathways and made a different choice.

Unwilling passenger

Our foster children are often passengers on such a trip. Two-year-old Vincent and four-year-old Bianca had a life changing moment, when their parents made a truly foolish decision. The children were in a car heading down the mountain, and their parents drove off the road. The family were legal immigrants from Mexico. At night, the parents put their children to bed, so they could go out to run errands. Their foolish decision wasn't leaving a sleeping three and four-year-old alone in bed. Their insane choice was leaving a fryer on, which set fire to the kitchen.

When the firefighters arrived, they found two children, but no adults. They called the police, who called social services. The children had no idea where their parents were. No one admitted to knowing the family and, even though there was no evidence of abuse, the children couldn't stay in what remained of the apartment. This was when CPS called us.

The police arrested the parents for child endangerment and it was some time before they avoided both prison and deportation, and were reunited with their children.

Vincent and Bianca's lives changed for a less obvious reason. They spoke only Spanish. Their parents only spoke Spanish, as did the other families who lived in the apartment block. A CPS placement worker called us at midnight that Sunday night and asked us to take the children. As we normally did, we asked for some information on the children. Given the circumstances, CPS only knew their names, and that they only spoke Spanish.

We speak no Spanish

I told the social worker we spoke no Spanish and she said she'd find a family who could. We returned to sleep until 2am, when she called back to say there were no Spanish speaking foster families, and could we please take these children. Sadly, for whatever reason, Dallas, Texas had few Spanish-speaking foster parents. I reminded her we spoke no Spanish, and couldn't see how the placement could work. At 3am, she called back pleading and begging, as there was nowhere and no one who would take them. At this point, we agreed and she promised they'd find a Spanish placement on the Monday morning.

The children arrived forty minutes later, in the clothes they had on when they left their house. We found some pajamas and put them to bed. This arriving with no possessions, no clothes, no favorite toys, no pacifier, no blankie, etc. was an unpleasant fact with our foster children. They came as "naked" as a newborn baby, even those who weren't newborns. Many had nothing at home either. With some, what they did bring weren't worth having. Drugs such as methamphetamine and cocaine leave a long lasting, powerful, smell on your clothes that stays for months.

Even getting the children to go to the bathroom, was complicated. I asked Bianca if she wanted to go to the bathroom. I took her into the bathroom and sat her on the toilet. She said "No quero el banyo." She wondered what I wanted her to do. It was 3:30am, I'd been woken three times by the phone calls, and I had no idea what she was saying either. We got them to bed and returned to sleep ourselves.

I've often wondered how it feels being a foster child, during those first few hours and days. Ann and I know about being a foster parent, during that same time. Foster children come into the foster care system with a lot of emotional baggage. The traumas that lead them to our home, most of us can't even imagine. Ann and I try to get information and each new story seems to be worse than the last one, in a never-ending escalation of horror.

Initially, we know nothing and have no idea what we're dealing with. All we know is their little spirit bubbles are filled with unimaginable negativity. Our method is to treat them as our own and start helping at once. Our plan of happiness states that they, and every one of us, are all children of God. They deserve the best we can offer. We try not to judge, even when it's the easiest thing to do.

Father's word is LAW!

Two of our children, Samir and Nakia, had come from a home where father's word was law. If you needed the bathroom, you needed permission. Unfortunately, asking was difficult and often dangerous.

We found this out the hard way when, thirty minutes after putting Samir to bed one night, I found him wandering in the hallway. I pointed back to the bedroom and he returned to his room without telling me why he was there. I was a bit too dense and didn't ask him. We found out the next morning, when his bed was wet. His dealings with his biological father made him decide it too dangerous to tell me what he wanted, or to ask permission. He thought wetting the bed would hurt less. He didn't wet the bed ever again, as we both learned from the incident. At least he didn't do what 4-year-old Evan did, which was to pee in the garbage can in the bedroom. It took me days to work out what the horrible smell was.

Even though they were our 70th and 71st foster children, Samir and Nakia proved to us that there is a lot we still need to learn. We didn't know how horrible their father was. We learned to ask this sort of question in the future.

With each foster child, we have thought they were surely the most abused children we'd ever had. Each time, we seemed to be wrong. Our actions and responses are based on our experiences and to Samir, the world was an unfriendly place. His spiritual bubble was permanently negatively charged. It would take a lot of time and effort to make it positively charged. He needed a lot of tender loving care. I have no idea if he ever received any after he left us.

Strangelove

Foster children tend to show love in the strangest ways. Some have learned from their parents how this works, or it doesn't. We have found they misbehave to see what we will do. Their plan of happiness is nearly blank, except for the idea of trusting no one.

We must prove we'll love them, no matter what. This doesn't happen overnight; the behaviors can go on for a long time, before they're know we won't kick them out. One reason Ann and I try to maintain positively charged spirit bubbles is to ensure we can engulf our children's negatively charged bubbles with love. and fill them with joy.

Hablos no Espanol

With Bianca and Vincent, the next morning we found some clothes for them, and performed pantomimes getting them fed. I left for work, leaving Ann to sort out the children. At work, I found a translation website on the Internet, and we used it to communicate with the children until they left. This wasn't the following morning, as there were no more Spanish speaking foster homes available on the Monday morning, than there had been on the Sunday night.

While they lived with us, Bianca came to think we were mad, in a hugely amusing way. We kept telling her in Spanish, we didn't speak Spanish. Her response was the obvious "yes you do, you're speaking Spanish right now." Her favorite title for us was Tonto or Tonta, which means silly, dumb or foolish.

Even with the language barrier, we quickly grew to love them and they us. When they left, they were more upset about leaving, than they'd been about coming to live with us in the first place. They were wonderful kids, who had not been abused. The memory makes me feel joyful, positively charging my spirit bubble.

Their parents knew the horror and life changing effect a foolish choice can bring. They were well educated, with all the necessary paperwork allowing them to stay and work in America. However, they had crossed a line, driven off the road and made a life changing decision, when they forgot to turn the power off on the fryer. They were lucky the firefighters didn't arrive to find dead children. They suffered through a lengthy period of hell, as they proved they shouldn't be deported, with or without their children. Happily, they did and several weeks later, the family was reunited. We hope they didn't make the same mistake again.

Not unique

Bianca and Vincent's parents are not unique in making dangerous, stupid mistakes. All of our children's parents have made stupid, dangerous errors of judgment that have also put their children's lives in danger.

We, you and I, are also capable of making stupid, dangerous choices. We may also find ourselves the victims of someone else's poor choices. How we deal with them will determine the path we follow in our lives. As a child, we also will find ourselves affected by choices which have been made by our parents. As a child, I moved house several times, because my parents were in the nursing profession and often the only promotional paths involved new hospitals in new cities. This required me and my siblings going to new schools and having to make new friends. We were given no choice in the matter; we were simply told that this was what was happening.

When the decisions are made for us, we still have a choice. Complain all the time, or get on with life. As no one really likes a complainer, our negative spirit bubbles will stay negative and others will do their best to stay clear of us.

Nothing changes, in my case we still moved house; I still lost friends; I still had to go to a new school and try to make new friends.

My foster children still came into the foster care system and 130 of them came to live with Ann and me.

This is a defining moment that makes us who we are. Everything is most certainly a trial bringing various type of mental and emotional pain. It's how we respond and deal with it that defines us.

I really don't hate dogs

Since I have begun training Dallas, our new Australian Shepherd, as a psychological service dog, I no longer dislike all dogs

Ann has noticed that, having him with me constantly as I have been working on socializing him, that I am benefiting as well. His training is different from the guide dog puppies we have trained. When he is in harness I allow him to check other people to see if they are feeling stress and then sit as close as he can, cuddling them. They have no choice but to hug and pet him back. He is filling people's spirit bubble with joy and happiness wherever I take him. This then fills my spirit bubble with joy.

Life as a foster child

The grand essentials to happiness in this life are something to do, something to love, and something to hope for.

You may wonder why I'm telling stories about some of my foster children. I'm doing so to show how life can be for those suffering unimaginable mental, spiritual and emotional pain caused by someone else making decisions and them paying the consequences. You may be able to relate to this. These consequences are much worse than going to a new school and needing to make new friends, although this is a part of it.

We may suffer physical, mental, spiritual or emotional pain caused by someone else's poor decisions. Or we may be suffering because we made the poor decision but we feel that no one else could have suffered as we are.

He's loud and weird

Only two of our six adopted children were old enough to remember life before they came to live with us. Elizabeth was 10 and Angelina 7. Elizabeth died four days after we completed the adoption, so I can't ask her. Angelina tells me she thought we were loud and I was weird. This impression of me is still the same, except now because she's a teenager.

It's not easy to put ourselves into the shoes of our foster children. It's very difficult to do so with biological children, so why would it be any easier with strangers?

Is everything sweetness and light? Not at all! Your life is turned upside down and you're told, not asked, you're going to live with another family. And you don't get to choose who. You may not have suffered physical pain, but you could have suffered mental, spiritual and emotional pain before now. You're possibly suffering from all three right now. Physical pain can cause all three of the other types.

88

Imagine

Imagine, if you can, you're a child who, for no apparent reason, is with a stranger in a cold office building at 2am, having been taken there by a police officer. You have no idea what's happening. The SWAT team, kicking your house doors in, woke you. They moved all the furniture, turned the beds over, looking for drugs, which they found. They arrested your brother, mother and grandparents, while your little brother and sister are sitting with you, in what they say is CPS.

Or, you came home from school to find a cop car at your house and strangers take you away, as if you were a criminal. Or, a teacher notices some bruises. Or, your parents get into a drunken brawl, and get themselves arrested. Or your mom shoots your dad.

Whatever the reason, you've done nothing wrong, yet you're sent to live with strangers, possibly with a different skin color and / or accent, with a bunch of children you take an instant dislike to, or who take an instant dislike to you.

Their lifestyle is nothing like you're used to. They have rules to obey, and you're used to doing what you wanted, when you wanted. They want you to go to bed at, what they say is a reasonable time, when you want to stay up all night and sleep until late afternoon, every day. They want you to eat the food they prepare for you and you prefer to eat each meal at McDonald's. You swear, you're sanctioned. Your parents swore constantly, so what's the problem?

They send you to a school full of preppies or gangsters, or whatever is the opposite of what you're used to. None of your friends lives anywhere near where you now live. You go to a new school, where you have no friends. Everything they teach is new.

Because you're a foster child, the other children and sadly the school officials treat you as if you were a child killer. If you step out of line one tiny bit, they come down on you, like a ton of bricks. You see other children who behave much worse than you do, yet they don't get into trouble. The other kids look at you funny and know you're strange. The stupid foster parents make you do stupid homework; your stupid parents didn't. They weren't even that interested if you ever went to the stupid school at all.

Stupid

You must learn all the stupid names of the stupid people who live in this stupid house. (They don't say stupid, they use or think swear words). You get to see your stupid parents once a week but only for one hour. They don't necessarily show up and, if they do, they're wasted, or they ignore you, or both. They split you and your brothers and sisters up, so you only see them once a week at these visits, when some other stupid foster parents bring them. You wonder why you can't see them more often and the stupid foster parents tell you, the stupid judge says you can't. You think they're lying, but there's nothing you can do.

It isn't hard to guess what's in the child's spirit bubble and it isn't joy. Most "only" have three of the four types of pain; mental, spiritual and emotional. A high number can also add physical pain.

Choices other people made

As foster parents, Ann and I have looked after children with all the dreadful problems caused by choices their mothers made during pregnancy. Some children have been born with so much alcohol in their systems they'd have been arrested for DUI; others with the horrible shaking a drunk, who is drying out, suffers. Others have been born addicted to cocaine, methamphetamine, heroin, crack or cocaine and have gone through the horrors of detoxification.

One of our foster children was on Methadone until they were 11 months old. If they ever decide to experiment with drugs, they may quickly get addicted. This is unfair, as it's a result of someone else's decisions. Nevertheless, they have to be careful around drugs.

Fetal Alcohol Syndrome

Their mother's selfishness has ruined these children's lives. There is no cure for the damage done to them. The National Institute of

Health (NIH) reports that, because it affects a person's ability to know the difference between right and wrong, as many as half of all teenagers arrested in the USA have Fetal Alcohol Syndrome (FAS). They can be naive, easily led and unable to make good value judgments. They're more likely to make poor choices. none have normal brain development.

Don't tell me alcohol and drug abuse doesn't affect me! If none has normal brain development; if they're making poor choices, my life is affected as well. If half the teenagers arrested have FAS, then half of teenage crime in the USA is caused by mothers-to-be who abuse alcohol! Government statistics shows 1/3rd of all crimes are committed by people trying to get money for their next drug fix.

Fourteen-year-old Adalyn's FAS problems and the issues caused by her mother's abuse of her in the womb were causing untold evils in her life. She had no moral standards to fall back on. She would get the phone numbers of truckers and give our number out, when we were on vacation. She'd try to sneak out the house at night. She had an attitude that got her into trouble at school and with her peers.

We all need to take responsibility for our actions, but, when the part of your brain that manages impulse control was damaged before you were even born; it can be hard to make good choices. She left us to go to a lock-down situation and probably went through another 4 or 5 foster homes, before she aged out of the system at 18 and had to look after themselves.

I know this is all horrendous. Unfortunately, nothing pleasant is what happens to abused children. All our babies have suffered because their mothers have abused alcohol, heroin, marijuana, cocaine, methamphetamine and a host of other drugs during their pregnancies. Many women have used them all while pregnant. The children suffer from the ghastly problems associated with drug abuse. The state only intervenes after the irreversible damage has been done, not before the damage begins.

Can you help?

Another reason I mention my children is to show that what you and I suffer may not be as bad as we believe. Although, they don't have to deal with our problems either, I would not swap. The main reason is to show how even horrendous mental, spiritual and emotional scars can be fixed and spirit bubbles charged with positivity. "All" it takes is tender loving care and a huge amount of time and energy. Another reason is letting others know the problems foster children deal with and have you consider helping.

I accept not all of us can be a foster parent. My plan of happiness didn't start with the idea of being one, but it finished off being a key part.

I joke the first requirement for being a foster parent is being certifiably mad. I have suggested to several of my friends they are already well on the way to meeting it. Some even have become foster parents.

Current government figures put the number of foster children adopted each year at about 50,000. This leaves approximately 112,000 children waiting to be adopted and a further 300,000 who are in the system hoping their parents get their lives in order. More than 20,000 age out each year. They are classed as adults, who no longer need any help. For many, if not all of them, this is not true. They have to start adulthood from an impossible position.

If you feel you can help, I would recommend you contact your local Foster Parent Association and inquire. If not, there is much you could do to help, when you find out someone is a foster child. You can also NOT do things when you find the other person is a foster child or used to be one.

Never assume we know the back-story

After a while, it becomes easy to recognize when someone has a negatively charged spirit bubble. The obvious response to these people would be to ignore them and assume they're zounderkites; nasty, unpleasant people. Because we make assumptions, many of us make this mistake. Some people do it, even when they know the back-story.

92

I want to fill my spirit bubble with joy. I want to fill my children's bubble with joy and happiness, despite the horrors they've suffered. All they want is love, so I show them love, transmitting joy and happiness from my spirit bubble to theirs by the things I do for and with them.

If you're not interested in being a foster parent, do at least take the time to wonder why a person, young or old, behaves the way he or she does. We may not be in a situation to intervene, but we can try to fill their spirit bubbles with joy and happiness. My method of pain management also works with those with negatively charged spirit bubbles. I am positive and I smile at others I pass. I ask them to smile and see their bubble positively charge. There will still be people who are zounderkites. We don't have to be one ourselves. We can be positive!

This story by Jean E. Mizer shows the opposite effect.

It started with tragedy on a biting cold February morning, I was driving behind the Milford Corners bus as I did most snowy mornings on my way to school. It veered and stopped short at the hotel, which it had no business doing, and I was annoyed, as I had come to an unexpected stop. A boy lurched out of the bus, reeled, stumbled and collapsed on the snow bank at the curb. The bus driver and I reached him at the same moment. His thin hollow face was white even against the snow.

"He's dead," the driver whispered.

It didn't register for a minute. I glanced quickly at the scared young faces staring down at us from the school bus. "A doctor! Quick! I'll phone from the hotel..."

"No use. I tell you he's dead." The driver looked down at the boy's still form. "He never even said he felt bad," he muttered, "just tapped me on the shoulder and said, real quiet, 'I'm sorry." I have to get off at the hotel.' That's all. Polite and apologizing like."

At school, the giggling, shuffling morning noise quieted as the news went down the halls. I passed a huddle of girls. "Who

93

was it? Who dropped dead on the way to school?" I heard one of them half whisper.

"Don't know his name; some kid from Milford Corners," was the reply.

It was like that in the faculty room and the principal's office "I'd appreciate your going out to tell the parents," the principal told me. "They don't have a phone, and anyway, somebody from school should go there in person. I'll cover your classes."

"Why me?" I asked. "Wouldn't it be better if you did it?"

"I don't know the boy," the principal admitted levelly.

"And in last year's sophomore personalities column I note that you were listed as his favorite teacher."

I drove through the snow and cold down the bad canyon road to the Evans place and thought about the boy, Cliff Evans, His favorite teacher! I thought. He hasn't spoken two words to me in two years! I could see him in my mind's eye all right, sitting back there in the last seat in my afternoon Literature class. He came in by himself and left by himself.

"Cliff Evans" I muttered to myself, "a boy who never talked." I thought a minute, "a boy who never smiled. I never saw him smile once."

The big ranch kitchen was clean and warm. I blurted out my news somehow. Mrs. Evans reached blindly toward a chair. "He never said anything about bein' ailing."

His stepfather snorted. "He ain't said nothin' about anything since I moved in here."

Mrs. Evans pushed a pan to the back of the stove and began to untie her apron.

"Now hold on," her husband snapped. "I got to have breakfast before I go to town. Nothin' we can do now anyway. If Cliff hadn't been so dumb, he'd have told us he didn't feel good."

After school, I sat in the office and stared blankly at the records spread out before me. I was to close the file and write the obituary for the school paper. The almost bare sheets mocked the effort. Cliff Evans, white, never legally adopted by stepfather, five young half-brothers and sisters. These meager strands of information and the list of D grades were all the records had to offer.

Cliff Evans had silently come in the school door in the mornings and gone out of the school door in the evenings, and that was all. He had never belonged to a club. He had never played on a team. He had never held an office. As far as I could tell, he had never done one happy, noisy thing. He had never been anybody at all.

How do you go about making a boy into a zero? The grade-school records showed me. The first and second grade teachers' annotations read "sweet, shy child;" "timid but eager." Then the third-grade note had opened the attack. Some teacher had written in a good firm hand: "Cliff won't talk, uncooperative. Slow learner." The other academic sheet had followed with "dull", "slow witted;" "low IQ" They became correct. The boy's IQ score in the ninth grade was listed at 83. But his IQ in the third grade had been 196. The score didn't go under 100 until seventh grade. Even shy, timid, sweet children have resilience. It takes time to break them.

I stomped to the typewriter and wrote a savage report pointing out what education had done to Cliff Evans. I slapped a copy on the principal's desk and another in the sad, dog-eared file. I banged the typewriter and slammed the file and crashed the door shut, but I didn't feel much better. A little boy kept walking after me, a little boy with a peaked, pale face; a skinny body in faded jeans; and big eyes that had looked and searched for a long time and then had become veiled.

I could guess how many times he'd been chosen last to play sides in a game; how many whispered child conversations had excluded him; how many times he hadn't been asked. I could see and hear the faces and voices that said over and over, "You're a nothing, Cliff Evans."

A child is a believing creature. Cliff undoubtedly believed them. Suddenly it seemed clear to me: When finally there was nothing left at all for Cliff Evans, he collapsed on a snow bank and went away. The doctor might list 'heart failure' as the cause of death, but that won't change my mind.

We couldn't find ten students in the school who had known Cliff well enough to attend the funeral as friends. So, the student body officers and a committee from the junior class went as a group to the church, being politely sad. I attended the services with them, and sat through it with a lump of cold lead in my chest and a big resolve growing through me.

I've never forgotten Cliff Evans nor that resolve. He has been my challenge year after year, class after class. I look up and down the rows carefully each September at the unfamiliar faces. I look for veiled eyes or bodies scrounged into a seat in an alien world.

"Look kids" I say silently, "I may not to anything else for you this year, but not one of you is going to come out of here a nobody. I'll work or fight to the bitter end doing battle with society and the school board, but I won't have one of you coming out of here thinking himself into a zero."

Most of the time, not always, but most of the time, I've succeeded.

I can't read the story without a lump coming into my throat. A movie was made of it, called *Cipher in the Snow,* and I cannot watch it without crying. One word that stands out to me in the story is the word "never". It's used 12 times, 11 times about Cliff Evans. This word should only be used when it indicates finality; when there's no possibility the statement it is attached to, can ever be wrong. I think the author is unfortunately right to overuse the word.

We can't know when the people we meet hurt so much, any simple act of kindness will help them. It's not clear if Cliff Evans was a real young man who died because no one cared, it is possible. If someone had communicated with him, had spent time and built him up, I'm sure Cliff Evans wouldn't have died. He died because his spirit bubble had no joy in at all. No one made any attempt to fill it with anything other than negativeness.

Here are a few suggestions to fill our spirit bubble with joy by filling other's spirit bubbles with happiness.

- *When we see a blind person with a guide dog, do not ignore them. They are blind not deaf. They'd probably appreciate talking to us.*

- *When we see a disabled person in a wheelchair talk to them as well as to the person pushing. They may not be able to stand up, but that doesn't mean they can't talk for themselves. They're probably as mentally sound as us, or anyone else.*

- *When a friend comes to talk to us about a problem, listen. Don't recount the time we had a similar or worse problem. Listening is a gift without compare. Many times, all they want is for somebody to listen. They don't want any advice, they want their feelings validated more than anything else. If we can listen to them, they will invariably have solved the problem themselves, by the time they have finished recounting their woes. There may be no solution to the problem, but I can guarantee if they know someone was interested enough in them to give them a listening ear, the problem doesn't seem as large.*

- *When a family member achieves something, congratulate them on that achievement. They could have come first, if they'd tried a bit harder, but so what? They achieved something, didn't they? There'll always be things that could be done better. Absolute perfection is only possible occasionally. Don't celebrate mediocrity, but praise what they did do.*

- *Apologize, even when we aren't necessarily in the wrong. Ask which is more important, being right or being in the right, doing the right thing?*

I could list more instances of where we can be positive and build others up, but I'm sure you can think of more yourself. The key is to be positive and we'll make a difference. We'll also find those we're kind to, may repay our kindness. We positivize their spirit bubble and they may do the same for ours. A positive spirit bubble makes it hard to concentrate on pain. It has gone nowhere, it's still there. We're ignoring it.

We need to do this even when others seem determined to be unpleasant. When we have, for example, just washed the dishes and someone comes along and tells us the dishes are still dirty. They then rummage through the pile of dishes until they find the one non spotless dish. This is the time when we need to be and stay positive because the other person most definitely has a negatively charged spirit bubble and we could be in danger of being overwhelmed.

Giving of ourselves

The ability to give of ourselves to others makes us a better person and the world a better place. It may even save the lives of people like Cliff Evans. Giving may involve money, but often it is a resource far more precious. Ourselves. Giving of that most precious resource, time, says far more than money ever can. If someone has broken down and is stuck at the road side, offering money isn't much help. Asking if we can help, may well be much more useful. Of course, with the world the way it is, it can be dangerous to do even this. But, assuming we aren't dealing with a mentally sick person, a lift to the nearest garage may well be appreciated. We may find it too risky to stop, and I'd be the first to agree our own safety comes first. How many times, though, have you been in a situation when that was nothing more than a convenient excuse? Only you can answer that, only you answer to your conscience. It doesn't matter what anyone else thinks.

As a young couple starting out in marriage, Ann and I were finding it difficult to make ends meet. In some situations, we felt we couldn't get the ends into the same room! Then someone offered to give us some money with the proviso we had to repeat the kindness to someone else. We have many times heeded that advice and passed it on, by helping other couples in dire straits. Whenever we have helped others with gifts of food, money or clothes, we've not suffered from doing so. In fact in many cases we seem to have been better off from doing so than we were before we started. This appears to be a law of the universe. If we need help, then help someone else first. Why and how this works, I don't know, all I know is that it does. We may not need to know how something works to make the decision to use it. A light switch is a simple example, giving to someone else and receiving more back in return is another.

Those who give and those who don't.

The following little article has no by-line, but it aptly defines the difference between people who give and people who do not. Those who are sel**fish** and those who are sel**fless.**

There are two seas in Palestine – one is fresh and there are fish in it. Splashes of green adorn its banks. Trees spread their branches over it and stretch out their thirsty roots to sip of its healing water. Along its shores, the children played when He was there. He loved it. He could look across its silver surface when He spoke His parables. On a rolling plain, not far away He fed five thousand people.

The River Jordan makes this sea with sparkling water from the hills so it laughs in the sunshine. Men build their houses near it and the birds build their nests. Every kind of life is happier because it is there.

The River Jordan flows on south into another sea.

Here is no splash of fish, no fluttering leaf, no song of birds, no children's laughter. Travelers choose another route unless on urgent business. The air hangs heavy above its waters, and neither man, beast nor fowl will drink.

What makes this mighty difference in these neighboring seas? Not the River Jordan. It empties the same good water into both. Not the soil in which they lie, nor the country roundabout.

The difference is that the Sea of Galilee receives but does not keep the Jordan; for every drop that flows into it another drop flows out. The giving and receiving go on in equal measure. The other sea is shrewder, hoarding its income jealously. It will not be tempted into generous impulses. Every drop it gets it keeps. The Sea of Galilee gives and lives. The other sea gives nothing; it is named "The Dead Sea." There are two kinds of people in the world. There are two seas in Palestine.

If we only take, we can be compared to the Dead Sea, never giving anything back. Which one do you feel you are?

This is another law of the universe. Those who don't give, not only don't get helped they seem to finish off with nothing. Another rule we may not like, but there is nothing to be done about. If you don't give, you don't get.

I know there are some people who take at the point of a sword or a gun. Most of these also seem to eventually finish off with nothing. This doesn't seem to be true of all people, but if we could see the lives of those we think don't have to pay, we would find them not to our liking. A few people, those who allow their lives to be ruled by their love of money, generally don't have friends who would stay around if the money went away. They are there because of their love of money not the rich person.

What do I give?

A couple of pages ago, I suggested some things we could do to make a difference. Here are a few others to consider as you decide how you're going to fill your spirit bubble with joy.

• *Visit the sick.*

- *Give sincere compliments, no matter what.*
- *Do someone a favor, even if they owe you one.*
- *Call and cheer someone up.*
- *Make a meal for people in a homeless shelter.*
- *Give a beggar or a tramp our small change.*
- *Pay it forward.*

Happiness and having a positively charged spirit bubble are achieved by choice, not by money, possessions or even necessarily by succeeding. Rich people can be unhappy and poor people can be happy. People who are successful in one area of life may be unhappy, because they are failing in another area.

Which is the right way?

On my journey down the mountain in Moab, I'm amazed we found our way across the desert, as we had no idea which way to go. The route we'd come wasn't clear, so I doubt we could have retraced our tracks. We looked for tire tracks and hoped that whoever had gone this way before, knew where to go. When we realized we were going the wrong way, we backed up. Several times, there were multiple distinct sets of tire tracks, branching off in different directions and no way of knowing which the correct ones were. We only knew I'd chosen correctly, when we eventually reached Moab.

Pain, whether mental, spiritual, emotional or physical, takes us down a road where we have little or no control, or idea where we'll finish off. My children have all learned they can be happy and pleasant when we're at the store and get a candy, or they can be a royal pain in the neck and have privileges removed. A question they ask a lot is, why? Why do they have to come to the store with us? What's wrong with them staying at home? Our answer is based on the idea of because we say so. We worry for their safety and being their parents we actually do know better, regardless of what they think.

When the reason you are "suffering" is because your mother made poor choices before you were born, it's harder to answer. You made no choices, she made them for you and they were all decisions that were best for her, not you. In fact, they were all very bad for you.

Deal with it!

When my children's buttons are pushed, they can find it hard to "deal with it". A word, phrase, smell, or sound triggers memories from their past and they occasionally lose it. My suggestions to help are humorous, like imagining the other person is a purple frog with yellow spots. When they speak, imagine they are on a lily pad being attacked by a dragon. The humor deflects the hurt.

When my pain buttons are pushed I have the same problem dealing with it. The choice is how I respond to the situation, not whether I have the pain. The no-pain road has washed out. I can do so cheerfully and, or I can be angry and irritable. I believe I'll be cheerful and do everything I can to positively charge and fill my spirit bubble with joy.

Tenacious or pig-headed?

Money can't buy you happiness, but it does bring you a more pleasant form of misery. (Spike Milligan)

Sometime in the future, around the time they find a cure for cancer and the common cold, someone may find a cure for RSD and other chronic pain conditions. And, (never begin a sentence with the word 'and', it annoys grammarians) there's nothing we can do about it.

I doubt anyone will find a way to stop mental, spiritual and emotional pain from occurring. It's not an good idea anyway, as we learn from our experiences even, or especially, the painful ones. It's not fair that we don't get the same amount of knowledge from good ones.

How do we find joy and ignore pain? This is where obstinacy becomes useful in doing so. Many people frown on this trait, but I've found it useful in turning pain into joy. The word means various things from pig headed, inflexible and unmanageable, to tenacious and strong-minded.

I am strong-minded

If I'm strong-minded enough, I *can* make some pain go away for a while. Imagine two levels, where the left one is the **amount** of pain we're in and the right one is the amount we can **handle**. With the right one higher, life is manageable. If the left one is higher, we have a problem. We only control the one on the right and it is here we need to be strong-minded. The amount of pain we're in pain is not something we can easily change. How we deal with it is.

103

Stubborn streak

Two of our foster children were obstinate, but not in a useful way. Aailuah had a large stubborn streak. This must have given her grandparents plenty of opportunity to test their disciplinary measures of hitting her and her sister with a vacuum cleaner hose. They also made the girls, who were three and two, squat next to the dinner table, for such heinous crimes as eating quickly, or speaking too loudly during a meal.

If Aailuah decided she didn't want to do something, we had to use our greater height and strength. One time, she wouldn't go beyond the line in the middle of the road and sat down, refusing to get up. The line was a "line in the sand", not to be crossed. At three and a half, even though she couldn't articulate this clearly, she made it obvious, here and no further. Luckily, the road was lightly used and Ann picked her up, before any cars came. I'm sure this stubbornness has continued and has caused both Aailuah and her mother a lot of grief over the years.

Keep on Walking

McKenzie also had a dominant personality, but she often made us smile with the way she behaved. Where Aailuah was willful and obstinate, McKenzie was obstinate in a withdrawn and introverted way. It was sad, but made for some fun moments.

She'd walk into walls and keep walking, believing she could walk through them. She'd decided she wanted to go that way, and no wall wasn't going to stop her. We were in a store and she walked into a huge bear of a man. Being up against his leg didn't slow her down one bit. She simply tried harder. I was initially too surprised to do anything. The man looked down at her and gave me an odd smile. I pulled her to the side and, like a wind-up toy, she took off as if nothing had happened. I shrugged my shoulders, smiled at the man, and followed.

After five months, Aailuah and McKenzie left us to return to their mother, who proved being deaf wasn't the problem her mother had claimed when she took the children off her. Them coming into care gave mother the opportunity to convince people she was a fit parent. If not for the social worker, they'd have gone home earlier. The worker was one of the few we have worked with who weren't interested in making the case progress and getting the children back home. She was a one-woman negativizer. She could make others feel down and depressed simply by being around.

Caseworkers

Most of our caseworkers have been wonderful people. The bad ones, such as this one, stand out in our memory. She didn't do what needed to be done and blamed either mother's deafness, or our refusal to cooperate. Neither statement was valid; we were more than willing to cooperate. She was incompetent and forgot to make appointments. If she made them, she'd forget to inform people of meetings. Several meetings had to be canceled, when she forgot to invite a deaf signer so mother knew what was happening. Ann knows how to sign in British Sign Language. In one of those many aspects of Murphy's Law, American Sign Language is completely different. As mother couldn't lip-read, such significant meetings were impossible.

We made sure we left nothing to the social worker, who was a zounderkite, and pushed and escalated the issue through successive levels of management at CPS, until the family was reunited. I'm not conceited enough to think only Ann and I could have helped the girls. Many other foster parents could have returned them to their mother. The fact is, we did and we're proud to have done so.

Obstinacy

The children set the standard against which we have compared all our later children. Their type of obstinacy isn't the type that helps us find joy through the pain. They fit the pig headed, inflexible and unmanageable end of the scale. Dealing with this stubbornness is hard on parents. I occasionally pretend I'm dealing with the Dr. Seuss characters Thing One and Two from The Cat in the Hat. I tell the child to do the opposite of what I want and warn them against doing so. It isn't so easy with adults, but little ones can be tricked into obedience, especially when they are praised for doing what we wanted. I do whatever I can to positivize their and my spirit bubbles.

Stubbornness is useful when managing pain. It takes a lot of effort, tenacity and being strong-minded to do so. We need to be like McKenzie in the way nothing can stop us. I don't recommend the illogical idea of expecting the mountain to move out of our way, but we should admire her tenacity. It's more than useful when trying to be strong-minded enough to carry on, to keep on walking, even when it hurts to do so. To keep on doing anything when everything hurts.

There are obstacles we cannot get past, without changing our current way of thinking. We have to be tenacious and show we want to change and the person we have to show is ourselves.

Reflection

Reflection is another useful tool. This is repeating and rephrasing what we heard. We might say "Let me make sure I understand, you're disappointed and upset your sister (whatever sister did)." We then validate their right to those feelings and ask for suggestions to correct the problem. Most people calm down when we do this, even children. The negative emotions seep out from their spirit bubbles, because they realize someone else cares enough about them to listen to them.

Distraction

Another useful psychological trick is distraction, where we change the topic and come back later to what we wanted them to do. With McKenzie, I'd point things out in a different part of the store and we'd look at it, without having to walk through the shelves or anything else.

At five, Olwen was as stubborn as Aailuah. One morning, she decided she didn't want to wear a certain shirt. It took me redirecting and distracting her, with invisible dragons eating her legs, to calm her down, before we arrived at school. She finds the dragons so silly she can't stop laughing. With pain, I accept what I can't do and concentrate on what I can. When I hurt, I stop and consider how to do things differently. If using my left arm and hand hurts, can I use my

106

right arm to do it? Or will I need to use both arms? I can't run to get something, can I get there by walking instead?

Control Room

Many of the things I have mentioned, including joy and obstinacy, are emotions which are handled by the mind part of the brain, the invisible internal part of us. The mind is in a secret part, the spiritual body, which no one ever sees. No one sees it, not even us, ever.

You may not be a religious person, I've no way of knowing, but you must agree the inner you, the part of us who looks out of our eyes and hears with our ears, is separate from the physical us. There are many words we could use, including chi, inner self, life force, soul etc., spirit fits best for me. If you feel the need to, you can substitute a different word. Our spirit is in control of our physical body, in the same way we drive a vehicle and, in the same way we take care of our car (or don't), our spirit takes care of our physical body. It also controls our spirit bubble. Our spirit uses our plan of happiness as a manual to decide how to behave and how to fill our spirit bubbles.

That can't be how I look and sound.

Our spirit often seems surprised at how the physical body looks. Even though we've seen ourselves in the mirror and heard ourselves speak every day of our lives, we're all surprised and often shocked, when we see and hear ourselves on a video. We don't look exactly the way we thought we did and can't believe we sound the way we do. This is true of us all, no matter how positive we feel about ourselves.

Modern technology has some wonderful gadgets. One is an adjustable magic mirror, which allows the user to change the way they look. Researchers on the TV show Horizon had volunteers use the mirror which was set to show the volunteer two-feet tall and ten-feet wide. They had to adjust the view, until the picture was correct. Everyone got it wrong, not greatly, but enough to be noticeable when compared to the "correct" view. Those with good self-esteem, made themselves better than the reality. Those with a poor self-image, made themselves worse.

Our spirit decides how we behave and our level of self-esteem. If it is small, insecure and inferior; regardless of how the physical body looks we'll behave small, insecure and inferior. Those with large, self-confident, self-assured spirits are larger than life, regardless of their physical stature. Even when handicapped in some way, the spirit can be in such control, the handicap is ignored or not obvious.

All self-help books are aimed at the spirit, because only it can change both the inner and outer person. Where the physical body is in charge there always seem to be problems with cravings and addictions.

Where is our spirit?

Where does our spirit live? No one, and I mean no one, has any idea. All we know is that when the body can no longer support life, our spirit leaves and isn't wherever it was. As no one knows, imagine our spirit is in a super control room, with hundreds of computer screens, organized into sections around the control room, a bit like in a science fiction star-ship.

Our spirit is sitting in the captain's chair. Computers control each section and cascade up to the master control program, then to us. We have billions of crew-members, or nanobots, at our command. They can do whatever we ask and act as messengers between the control room and all parts of our brain and body. We're happy to let the brain automatically manage the minute-to-minute control of most functions and information coming in and going out, using programs we've created since we were a baby. This is good, because we receive millions of bits of information each second.

The computer industry uses a method of figuring out processor speeds; Millions of Instructions per Second (MIPS). The fastest recorded multi-core computers with 750,000 cores are rated at 10 trillion MIPS. Neurologists suggest the human brain is faster.

The Limbic System

The main screen, through which virtually every input message comes into our brain, is the **Thalamus** screen in the **Limbic System** region. It's the switchboard of our brain and responsible for signal relaying and prioritization.

Our sensory systems receive far more data than we can use. The thalamus condenses data which the higher brain sections can manage. It also has connections to the other parts of the limbic system. In our control room model, each has its own computer system and screen, all connected to the master control system.

- *The hippocampus manages memory.*
- *The cerebellum controls muscle function.*
- *The amygdala regulates emotions, controls friendship, love and affection, the expression of mood, fear, rage and aggression.*
- *The hypothalamus deals with emotions, pleasure, rage, displeasure and sleep.*
- *The cingulate gyros handles emotional reaction to pain.*
- *The nucleus accumbens and Ventral Tegmental area releases dopamine.*
- *A small finger-sized control center, found at the base of the brain, called the reticular activating system (RAS) sorts and evaluates incoming data. It filters all incoming information and acts as a receiver for information tagged as important.*

There are 100's more brain areas and each brain area has many other functions, but we'll close the neurology 101 class here.

Aren't those names wonderful though? The definitions don't necessarily improve our knowledge. For example, the Merriam-Webster dictionary definition for the nucleus accumbens is: "a nucleus forming the floor of the caudal part of the anterior prolongation of the lateral ventricle of the brain." They use words such as anterior, instead of in front of; caudal, instead of behind of; and lateral, instead of the side, so lesser mortals have no idea what they're talking about.

The Pre-Frontal Cortex

The only other brain area we need to look at is the bit behind our foreheads, the Pre-Frontal Cortex or PFC. It has many bi-directional connections with the limbic system and oversees abstract or theoretical thinking, thought analysis, and regulates behavior. This includes handling conflicting thoughts, making choices between right and wrong, and predicting the probable outcomes of actions or events. Simplistically put, it's seems to be where our conscience lives.

The PFC governs social control, such as suppressing emotional or sexual urges and handles taking in data through the body's senses and deciding on actions. As you can see, it's a hugely important part of our brain and my candidate for qualities such as consciousness, general intelligence, and personality. Our spirit uses it to override programming in other brain areas. For example, the section responsible for eating, receives a message from the stomach; the hunger programs take control and instruct the body to find food. There's no link to the outside, and no concern over where the food comes from. The program might instruct the body to beg, steal or borrow some. The PFC makes sure we follow the rules and regulations, the moral standards by which we live. This is where and when our spirit uses our plan of happiness. We have decided to diet and the spirit will override the hunger programs. It will make the body wait to eat until the next meal time, or go for food more nutritious than the piece of chocolate.

There are some situations where the physical body must be in control. The most obvious is when we need to go to the bathroom. If we need to go, we'd better stop whatever we're doing and go to the bathroom. This fact is true for everyone. If your bladder or bowel needs to be emptied they are in control of everything.

Tickle our amygdala

Remember the two levels? The spirit controls the right one, how much pain we can stand. The left one is the amount of pain we're in, over which we have no control, other than with medication.

In the same way we use computers, even though we know little to nothing about the way they work, I believe we don't need much more information on the brain parts we need to use to be able to increase the right-hand level.

We'll start with the amygdala. Let's make ourselves feel a little better, right now by tickling it. No surgery is needed, which is good because our amygdala is a couple of inches inside our brain.

Inside our skull, where an imaginary line from the inner side of our eye and a line from the front edge of our ear would meet, are our two amygdalae. They are the shape of an almond (amygdala in Latin), so visualize two almonds. Imagine you have a feather and tickle the front of these almonds. Visualize the tickling sensation and you should feel a large rush of positive emotions, have happy peaceful emotions and you may even laugh. We have positively charged our spirit bubble.

Create a permanent program, an application. Have your spirit use the limbic system screens and load the app. You will feel those happy feelings. Tenacity becomes useful, if it doesn't seem to be working. Don't quit until you succeed, because it does work.

A second brain trick is a **thalamic cortical pause**. This is pausing, taking no impulsive action, and thinking through the implications of what we're about to do. When we are in any amount or type of pain, it allows us a moment to stop the negative response we're about to make.

There are other brain tricks we could do, to help with pain, but I have found shutting the pain gate, which we'll discuss later, and holding it shut, tickling my amygdala and using the thalamic cortical pause, work in most situations. My spirit bubble is quickly and efficiently positively charged.

It is possible that my spirit bubble is positively charged and yet for some reason the pain I am in is higher than I can manage. It doesn't happen too often, but I'd be lying if I said it never happened.

She Chose Poorly

*Happiness is a perfume you can't pour on others without getting a few drops on yourself. (**Og Mandien**).*

If we're happy, we bring happiness to others. A butterfly fluttering past on a warm and sunny day can make us feel good. We can make others feel good by smiling at those we pass. Smiling automatically makes us feel good as well. We fill our spirit bubble with happiness and it radiates to others.

In the movie, Easter Parade, Fred Astaire wants to see whether men will turn and look as Judy Garland walks down a street. He makes her walk a few feet in front of him to see what effect she has. Initially she turns no heads, and then all the men who pass are turning and looking back. Astaire is amazed, but is unaware Garland is pulling faces. I'm not suggesting we do this as we go places, but when we choose to smile it makes both us and the other person feel better.

Consequences

Consequences always follow actions and they can be unpleasant. Our ability to fight pain, find joy and positively charge our spirit bubbles is, in a significant way, controlled by the consequences of all our actions.

Kalyn came into care when police arrested her mother for drug dealing. She was selling drugs to pay for her own habit and automatically lost custody of her daughter. Kalyn was a week from her second birthday, and celebrated with us, instead of her mother. She is six months younger than Matthew and five months older than Emily, she fitted in with no difficulty. Kalyn was a beautiful, healthy, and intelligent two-year-old little girl, with an unconventional hairstyle. Mother had decided to dye her hair blond to disguise her. She was unclear if she wanted to hide her from CPS, or from Kalyn's father. Unfortunately for Kalyn, her mother had no cosmetology skills and she finished off with a strange streaky style. After a couple of months, her hair returned to light brown.

We already knew that one family member falling into drugs, alcohol and the seedier side of life, doesn't mean the rest of their family will. Kalyn's mother was the black sheep of the family. Her aunt couldn't have been more different.

When mother was arrested again, the family decided enough was enough and called DCFS. Kalyn was her 7th child and she was obviously going to do no more for number 7 than she had for the other 6. After a couple of weeks, Kalyn's aunt decided she had to step up to the plate. She started the process of taking legal custody of Kalyn and the baby moved in with them. The transition was an exciting process, as Kalyn already knew and loved her aunt. Mother's poor choices eventually worked out well for her little one. She made no effort to change, so Kalyn moved to live with a family who loved her and chose to make her their own. She was too young to realize she needed a forever family and yet she found one. She no longer had to deal with what her mother was doing. Her tiny spirit bubble was filled with joy not pain.

Kalyn is someone who had no control over the life changing decisions made for her. Fortunately, she had an aunt who didn't give the normal "not my problem" response. She could easily have argued her sister needed to get her life in order. She didn't. She could have argued Jalyn didn't need her help or that someone else should do something. She didn't. She could have argued she had too much pain to deal with already. She didn't do that either. She saw a need and met it. As a result, she added a little girl to her family, a little girl who had a huge need. She wasn't thinking of her own needs and the extra work that an extra child would bring to her family's life.

I don't care

Unlike her sister, the loss of her child didn't bother the mother. She could now continue her hedonistic lifestyle without needing to take care of her child. Her plan of happiness only held selfish actions. The only role fully defined was the "me" role. She made poor decisions based on having the pleasure pathways in her brain permanently on, regardless of the horrible effects this had on her physical body. I'm not too sure what her spirit bubble is filled with, but it's nothing positive, because she is a zounderkite. As she was only 31, it is likely that Kalyn was not her last child.

Choices

All decisions including good ones have consequences. I found how simple good choices can result in negative results, as I drove past a stationary police car. A truck passed me doing 85mph in a 60mph zone, causing my little car to shudder in his wake. The police car took off in pursuit. I watched him in my rear-view mirror, as I assumed he was after the truck and I wondered how long it would take him to catch up. I was surprised when I was pulled over instead. He'd seen me watching him in my mirror and pulled me over, because he thought I had something to hide.

I didn't and so he simply did a cursory examination of my car. I could have complained about his stopping me and made a lot of noise about wasting my time and ask why he wasn't stopping the truck, which was breaking the law. Instead, I chose to be polite and helpful. The policeman made one choice he regretted. For some reason, he decided to look in the back of my car, and asked me to open the hatchback. I did and he peered into the dark interior. It was late, dark and we were in the middle of nowhere. He got a huge shock, as our black and white pet collie dog barked loudly at him. He jumped back, and in a frightened voice told me to go. I'm sure the next time, he checked there were no animals in the car he was checking in the dark.

Change of underwear?

I often wonder whether he needed to change his underwear. I ask this because of something that happened while working at a large chemical facility. One day, I was thumbing through the safety reports, when one caught my eye. A crane jib had snapped while moving a multi ton piece of equipment which had fallen to the ground with a tremendous bang. Later in the report, there was an incident where a worker had gone home to change his clothes. There was a familiar looking related accident number, so I thumbed back through the report to the broken crane jib. The equipment had fallen next to the worker and he'd soiled his clothes from the shock of 10 tons of metal hitting the ground so close to him.

The policeman based his decision upon earlier experiences he'd had when following traffic. He'd stopped other drivers, who'd watched him the way I was, and he'd found they had some reason not to want to stop. In this instance, he chose wrongly. Had he kept on chasing the truck, he'd have stopped someone who was breaking the law, instead of being scared out of his wits. His spirit bubble was probably filled with some emotional and mental pain. I bet the next driver he stopped dealt with an angry policeman.

Long-term consequences

Whenever I've done something really stupid, my evil fairy Godmother ensures something physically unpleasant occurs to make sure I remember the result. My own Murphy's Law says if it can go wrong, it will and will leave lasting discomfort.

For example, my top ribs are not connected properly to my breastbone and every so often, I stretch and have them pop back into place. This hurts, both when they pop out and when I pop them back. I damaged my sternum in 1975, at a beach party at Tynemouth in the Northeast of England. A beach party is exactly what it says, a party on the sea shore, in this case, the North Sea. Each year, our church organized a party for all the youth. I was 19 and had recently moved to the area, so didn't know many people yet. This didn't stop me from being a tease and a prankster.

Pig's head

The best prank I pulled involved a freshly killed pig. I acquired the head at a local abattoir one lunchtime, took it back to work, and had a lot of fun with it. I put it on top of a cabinet in my office and everyone tried to convince their secretaries to come see me. Those who did open the door came face to face with a large pig's head.

I delivered it to a friend's apartment, in the middle of the night, with the help of two other guys who lived there. It can be frightening to wake up because the phone is ringing and, on your way to the telephone, trip over a dead pig's head. The prank worked perfectly and is still remembered and discussed 25+ years later as the ultimate prank.

Annoying the girls

At the beach party, I was an annoyance to the girls, who really didn't mind me annoying them. At one point, two tried to bury me in a hole they'd dug. They picked me up, carried me a couple of hundred feet up the beach, dropped me in the hole, and tried to bury me with the sand. I easily avoided this fate and got up to continue being a pest. I don't recall why another person and I picked up a girl and carried her out into the sea. Well I do remember why, I think that much is obvious. What I don't recollect is how I had the less appealing and more dangerous end. The Northeast of England has many miles of beautiful beaches dotted with the ruins of castles. Unfortunately, the sea is constantly cold. In winter, about 43F and in summer 63F, so playing in the water is always a bracing experience. She kicked and squirmed and eventually managed to free one foot and kicked me, right in the middle of my chest. I dropped her other foot and she squirmed free and ran back to the beach. I fell to my knees and groaned, before staggering back to the beach and the warmth of the fire. I couldn't complain about the damage, or admit a girl had caused me pain. All these years later, it still hurts.

If I was playing victim, reliving the story would make my chest hurt, it doesn't. It hurts no matter what. I choose to remember the fun of the party and my spirit bubble fills with joy. There's no room for pain. Nowadays, any one of my daughters, daughters-in-law, or granddaughters is more than willing to try to inflict lasting pain on me, generally for embarrassing them. One has decided she should pull the

116

hairs from my arm. It almost has me pausing before teasing her. Almost! It's painful, but, well!

Choices can't be unmade

My sternum is cracked and my ribs hurt constantly, because I decided to throw a girl into the sea in 1975. That choice can't be unmade. She kicked me hard in the chest, I could spend a lot of time, and effort complaining it's her fault I hurt. This is true, but I must take responsibility for the consequences as they affect me. If I can't, I'll spend my life playing the victim game and walk around with a negatively charged spirit bubble, as well as a sore chest. The sore chest is no longer negotiable.

There may be many people we need to forgive when something causes us pain. As hard as it is, we cannot move on until we do. There are no easy answers for me to give on how to do it, so I won't. I do know that I must carry on regardless, even when the other person won't apologize and then says and does more unpleasant things. This is even harder to forgive, but unless we want to have negatively charged spirit bubbles, we have no choice.

How we deal with forgiveness is another way we define ourselves. If we do something wrong to someone else, we need to ask for forgiveness. If we are the person who has been wronged we are the one who needs to give forgiveness.

Forgiving ourselves

Often the hardest thing to do is to forgive ourselves. For some strange reason, it's harder than forgiving others. We feel we deserve whatever is happening to us. I was driving the car when we had the accident, or I've been "naughty" and therefore merit it.

Others can make life worse by telling us the same thing. Karma, or God, is punishing **you** and if **you** hadn't done (whatever it was), **you** wouldn't be being punished now (with whatever is happening now). **You** weren't caught, but if **you** had been, **you'd** be in prison.

117

A person who steals can be sent to jail or prison or given a community order, but not **you**, **you** got away with it. But, **you** didn't really, did **you**? Because now **you** are being made to pay for **your** sins. If this were true, I must have had a very sinful life. None of which I can remember. Your belief that **you** deserve it all means **I** must deserve it.

Dreadful things can happen to good people

Terrible things happen to us all, at some time in our lives. None of us is immune. It may be no more than stubbing our toes, or using our shin to find things in the dark. It may be major, such as parents dying, spouse dying or worst of all, a child dying. We may lose our job and take some time to find a new one. The list goes on and on, terrible things can happen to any of us. They can just be dreadful or we can realize they give us the opportunity to learn and to grow.

As well as giving us a tough time, life constantly brings us good things. We need to concentrate on these and do our utmost to be positive. Bad things happen and we must learn to accept them, along with the good things.

There is no law of God, the universe, or anything else, which insists we're punished for what we've done in the past, once we have repented of them. Repentance has several steps and is necessary if we want to feel better about ourselves.

(1) Admit we did wrong.
(2) Feel sorry for what we did
(3) Ask for forgiveness
(4) Right the wrong
(5) Don't repeat the wrong

The final step is to forgive ourselves. If society needs us to, we may have to make restitution by going to jail, paying fines, community service, making repayment.

Once we've done this, we've paid our debt. Why should we be punished with psoriasis, RSD, or by becoming allergic to gluten? The fact I recently slipped on ice at the front of my house, hurting my elbow, head and shoulders is unrelated to anything I've done, or not done in the past. Except, had I removed the ice from the bottom of the steps after clearing the other steps, there would have been no ice to slip on. This, however, isn't karma.

To repeat, we are mistaken, if we think undesirable, unpleasant things happen to us because we are in some way evil. This doesn't happen to people who are evil. So why should it happen to those of us who aren't? This isn't a religious concept, it's a fact of life. There is no link between how good, bad or ugly we are and whether undesirable or unpleasant things happen to us.

Forgiving others

There is a group of people I constantly have to forgive; those closest to me. They cause me emotional, spiritual and mental pain and the worst part is they aren't doing it purposefully, or with any spite. Those of us with invisible, constant, chronic pain know it's impossible for others to know how it feels. Please believe me when I tell you, that when **you feel at your worst**, this is how I feel **when I'm doing well**. It's something you can't understand, unless you've also suffered from a full body chronic pain condition. But that's ok.

I find myself constantly forgiving others for forgetting I won't get better. They don't realize I'm simply happy, or rather, my spirit bubble is positively charged and I'm ignoring the pain. I can only suppose they believe that if they were in as much pain as I say I am in, they would not be as happy as I appear to be.

Service Fatigue

RSD, Fibromyalgia and all other chronic pain conditions are permanent conditions. Most people are happy to help until the problem resolves itself, the body gets fixed. People, even family members, become tired of helping when there is no end, when the pain stays.

Everyone who has suffered from a hidden condition has been on the receiving end of service fatigue. The definition causes it – it's hidden. No one can see the pain I am suffering from. There are no visible conditions, no plaster casts, no noticeably damaged body parts, missing limbs, etc. etc.

I have horrible pain which is invisible. There are surgery scars in various places, but they are all hidden. Both of my ankles, knees and hips hurt, so it's impossible for me to limp.

As there is no visible proof, it is easier for people to believe there is nothing wrong and to stop offering help. They are suffering from service fatigue, where they are tired of giving service because it has been going on for so long. I find myself needing to forgive people daily. It's essential I do and I'm glad I can. I'mnot glad that I have to, just that I have the ability.

To stay a victim, don't forgive.

Remember, to stay a victim, don't ever forgive yourself or others. This will ensure your spirit bubble is dark and full of negativity and there's no way we can help ourselves, or others. We must have a positive mental attitude (PMA), especially about ourselves. Forgiving ourselves is essential. We can't excuse what we did, but must remember our past mistakes guide, not define us. We're supposed to learn from our mistakes, not become them.

We can't fix them, as there is no returning; we can only learn from them. We may not have known better when we made the mistake. Now we do. We are **entitled** to have a positively charged spirit bubble. We must make positive choices even when we feel negative. A positive attitude makes it so much easier to do so, so be positive!

He doesn't stop, he can't be in pain!

One question I constantly hear is why don't I stop? Why keep on keeping on when if [the other person] was in as much pain as I claim to be in, they couldn't. They'd give up and stay in bed all day.

If I had the choice of doing nothing, I might. I probably wouldn't, but I don't have that choice. My entire body hurts, front, back and sides and everything in between. For some reason, sitting and lying down hurts more than standing does. Of course, standing quickly gets tiring and I must sit, which starts the cycle of hurting.

I don't stop hurting, ever. This, however, doesn't mean I should quit. Unfortunately, to make it hard for me, I must deal with other people's assumptions about me, which seem to go like this.

- *Pain is the body's defense system to stop us using the body part in need of repair.*
- *If we ignore the pain, we could do lasting damage.*
- *We use medications to lower pain until the body has repaired the traumatized part.*
- *He has used pain pills for 17+ years. The broken bits surely must have repaired by now.*
- *They've adopted 6 children, how can he still be in pain?*

Using these assumptions, someone who claims to be in pain, long after the traumatized part has repaired, must be, at best, telling lies. If X-rays, CT scans, MRIs show the affected part is okay, how can there be pain?

They've no idea what I'm talking about, or interest, when I say that vasoconstriction and adrenaline causes the pain. It's hard when for the past ten+ years, they have lived in the same community and I have complained of being in constant chronic pain the whole time.

You remember how when they first moved in, you helped them. Then a year later and every year since, they keep asking for help. When will they get better and stop asking? When the answer is never, service fatigue sets in.

I have no choice but to accept they aren't being purposefully mean and nasty to me, when they make these negative assumptions. I must act as if they aren't unpleasant and unhelpful and forgive them, even when nothing of what they are saying is remotely correct. I have no idea how to stop people making assumptions about me and my pain. All I know is to keep acting as if they are **not** and keep forgiving.

121

Fighting Pain Finding Joy

Some pain I deal with comes from trying to help my children deal with the horrors in their lives. I am in pain from all the traumas I deal with. I am also in pain as I try to help my children deal with their pain. The hard thing for me is having enough positive energy in my spirit bubble to be able to force the negative energy out of their bubbles. Not forgiving fills mine with negativity. I need a fully positively charged bubble, so we go around in a circle of needing to act **as if**.

If I do everything I possibly can to keep my spirit bubble filled with joy, I have a much better chance of overwhelming other peoples negatively charged spirit bubble instead of allowing theirs to overwhelm mine.

Having Children

Happiness consists of not having, but of being; not of possessing, but of enjoying. Man is the CREATOR of his own HAPPINESS.   (David O. McKay)

A big choice, which has been made made billions of times on planet earth, is to have children. That first baby pitches every new parent into completely unknown territory; we have no real idea what to expect. Or, if we think we do, we're still unprepared for what happens. We believe others are unprepared, we, the brilliant examples of humanity we are, will have no problems at all. Our spirit bubbles overflow with optimism and joy at the thought of how wonderful our baby will be and how we'll be the parents used as the perfect example in all the parenting books.

Sometimes life starts out wonderfully and we get a child who behaves as we expected. They're quiet, don't complain and behave in the same way we believe we did as children. We begin to think we're brilliant at this parenting game and decide it's time for number two.

Number two can be the same as number one. Most often, Mother Nature is leading us on, so she can deliver the sucker punch with number two. It may take a few weeks to notice and realize this time will be different. This one is different from the first one.

Is the baby called Damien or Carrie?

For Ann and I, a social worker asking us how the baby is doing, has been the catalyst for the child to change into a completely unexpected and, occasionally, a little scary monster. You may remember the horror movies, The Omen and Carrie, where the devil possesses the main characters. For many foster parents, the shorthand description for a difficult child is Damien or Carrie. Any other foster parent knows exactly what we mean and needs no further information.

This is where being a parent can become incredibly hard and many parents falter. 60% of foster parents quit within the first year and a further 20% in year two. When their license comes up for renewal, they don't bother.

We've noticed more children have come into care on days when life is stressful. When the weather's hot, as it is during school summer break, more children come into the foster care system. Why? Because their parents cannot cope! Some nights, DCFS in Dallas have had 50 babies they were searching for foster homes for. Once all the foster homes were full, they sent the babies to homeless shelters. Some were newborns!

Instead of being the center of attention, they go somewhere no one really cares about them. They begin life with spirit bubbles filled with pain. Even though we've only been able to help a few, Ann and I have been able to help some.

Poor parental decisions

All foster children are living somewhere other than at home, because of choices made by their parents. The choices may have been made many years earlier or recently, or both. Deena, Debbie, Daisy and Danielle came to live with us because Mom had reached the end of her tether and could no longer cope. They lived in a two-room shack, with no running water and no electricity. Unbelievably, there are towns in the USA, where this is still common. Without electricity, there was no air conditioning and during summer, where the temperature stays over 100F (38C) for weeks, it was unbearable. Mother walked with her children, two-year-old twins, a 10-month-old and a newborn, the couple of miles to the nearest town. She walked into the DCFS office and told the social worker she couldn't manage her children. She suggested they'd be better off living somewhere else and left. Having met her, I know how hard this decision was. Her spirit bubble was bursting with sadness over the decision she felt compelled to make, but she couldn't continue. The conditions in which she lived with her four baby daughters were impossibly hard

Abusive choices.

When alcohol and drug abuse are involved, the choices are all bad. As with the symptoms of RSD, the list of abuses is depressingly long. Children have suffered at the hands people who should have been giving them love. Many have suffered multiple types of abuse.

Some of our children have looked out the window to see what was swinging in the breeze. They were shocked and traumatized to see it was their stepfather, who had hung himself on the tree in the yard, after losing a fight with mother's current boyfriend over visitation rights. Some came to us with no clothing, others in pajamas because they had no other clothes. The heads of one itched intolerably, because she had lice infestations so bad we could see and count them.

As well as being born with fetal alcohol syndrome, or born addicted to cocaine, crack, methamphetamine or heroin at birth, some as young as two have been beaten so often, they're frightened of everything. A raised voice telling the dog to stop barking, because the doorbell has sounded, will cause them to become hysterically frightened. Some were beaten even for minor misdeeds. Tanis would burst into tears and sit there, cowering in fear, because she'd broken a crayon, or torn a piece of paper she was drawing on.

Others were sexually abused by their fathers, brothers, uncles, grandfathers, even random men, their mother invited into the house. A man, who wants to protect them, instead of hurting them, is confusing.

Some of our little girls have gone to school in their much older brother's cast off clothing.

Some children were so frightened of their biological fathers they couldn't even look at him on visits and screamed hysterically, when made to go into the same room as him. Others have pretended to fall asleep, as we entered the CPS office and stayed that way for the whole visit. Some children were woken up by exploding "flash bangs" and rousted from bed, by men wearing flak jackets with the letters SWAT.

Some have been shaken so badly, their brains have effectively exploded. A few newborns were critically ill and in pediatric intensive care for three months, yet their parents never visited them, except to

125

ask the nurse why they were treating them, as "they'd just be retards".

A two-year-old was stapled to a door and left there to cry for hours. A one-year-old would bang on a door and insist we "open this <bleeping> door." A seven-year-old, who was unable to tell us their last name and not because they were shy. The list goes on and on.

I know I've filled your spirit bubble with some mental, emotional and spiritual pain, as you process the horror my children have suffered through. As I said earlier, I'm telling their stories to show the countless ways we can find ourselves in pain and to prove there are countless ways of fighting pain and finding joy. To show this is true, let me fill your bubbles with some positive stories about these same children.

Let's do Christmas

Even though someone making a wrong choice is the reason all our foster children came to live with us, Ann and I have taken responsibility and done what we can to make life easier for them. We help them fight the pain, which may be physical, mental, emotional, or spiritual, or a combination of them all, and find joy. They can fill their spirit bubbles with this joy.

Being part of our family seems to have done this for most of them, and with some stunning exceptions I won't be talking about, have decided to fit in as if they'd been with us from the beginning.

Five-year-old Baylee and her eight-year-old sister Alyssa had done so, after initially having a tough time fitting into our life style, particularly with the number of people who came to our house. They assumed any gathering was a party and, as their religious beliefs told them they couldn't go to parties, they needed to sit in their room and not join in with us.

They told us they couldn't celebrate Christmas with us. A trip to Silver Dollar City in Branson, Missouri at Thanksgiving made them change their minds. Silver Dollar City is a Victorian Era theme park. There are all the modern rides and attractions, but all the staff dresses in Victorian clothes. At Christmas time, they have a five story Christmas tree with millions of lights. We can go on a steam train and visit with Grandpa, who tells the Nativity story. There are Christmas singers, carolers, Christmas plays and a huge attraction called Bethlehem Revisited, which acts out the Nativity. You can play with the animals in the stable and walk around a representation of Bethlehem at the time of Jesus.

It didn't take long for the girls to decide they should celebrate Christmas with us. Their spirit bubble filled with happiness and joy at the thought. We don't distinguish between our biological children, our adopted children and our foster children, so Christmas that year was joyful fun for us all. We had seven children to celebrate with, Simon, Andrew, Amy, Elizabeth, Matthew, Ben and Baylee. Ann's parents were also there, visiting from England.

After Christmas, the courts honored the biological father's request for custody and sent Baylee and Alyssa to live with him. Their mother was neither able, nor willing, to get herself sorted out, so she lost custody. This was a bittersweet experience for us. The girls were leaving to live with their father, a perfect result in the foster care world. We care for them, while the parents resolve their problems.

The only problem is the hole left in our heart. Before getting into the car with the social worker, Baylee turned to Ann and asked, "I'm sad to leave, will it be all right if I cry?" Ann replied, "It'll be Ok, because as you're driving down the driveway, crying, I'll be standing here crying as well." The driveway at our house was one hundred yards long, so the drive was a long one. We were happy they went with their father, yet sad to see them go. An example of joy and sadness occurring together. We had to choose which stayed and after the initial moments when our spirit bubbles were full of sadness, not joy, we decided to concentrate on the positive side of them going home.

Dante

I had a funny experience with Baylee. One of our cats managed to get its claws caught in our Berber carpet and ripped a six-inch wide channel for forty feet across two rooms. This irritated me, as it had also recently taken to using the sofa as litter tray. I banned all three cats from the house and joked that, as Dante's divine comedy only named nine circles or levels of hell, the cats were obviously from the tenth level. One, the best behaved and friendliest, went missing not long after. We assumed some wild animal had killed him. He'd recently lost a fight with a raccoon and had the claw marks on his back as battle scars.

We were planting flowers and Baylee came to watch. With one plant, I dug a deep hole and she asked if I was trying to find Tiger. I'd no idea what she meant and asked how I'd find him in a hole in the garden. She reminded me I'd said cats were from the tenth level of hell and assumed I thought Tiger had gone there. We eventually found his remains in the horse's water trough.

Mom!!! Dad!!!

We saw Baylee and Alyssa several times after they left. We were in a mall when we heard "Mum! Dad!" being shouted. As all parents do, we looked around and noted all our children were present, so we ignored the shouting. The shouting continued and we turned around to see Baylee and Alyssa running as fast as they could towards us from the other side of the mall.

A few minutes later, their father, who we hadn't previously met, caught up and looked at us quizzically, as we hugged his daughters. We explained who we were and he was then friendly. We hugged and chattered for some minutes, until their dad could convince them to come with him.

Another time, I was heading into a store, when I saw the girls and waved and smiled at them. An older woman with them looked at me with an angry stare and hastily pushed the girls into the store. I shrugged my shoulders; I didn't know her either. A minute or so later, the woman came running out the store, again pushing Alyssa and Baylee ahead of her. She told me the girls had explained who I was and she'd returned to apologize for her impolite behavior. She thanked me for caring for and loving her granddaughters, through a challenging time in their lives. We chatted for a few minutes, I hugged the girls and they left again. My spirit bubble fills with joy each time I recall or retell tell these stories, and pain and depression go away for a while. I can do more when I feel good.

Poor choices and good choices.

Some choices are good and some poor, but there are always consequences. We may suffer the consequences ourselves, either positive or negative. At other times, someone else must pay for our decisions.

Our foster children's parents all made a whole series of poor choices and their children must pay the consequences. The hard part for me, as a parent, is despite this, the children need to learn that their own choices have consequences, for which they must pay. What their parents did to them is unfair, but in the same way as it's unfair I have RSD, they must make good choices with what they have. Our job is to praise them for good choices and help them deal with the consequences when they don't. Remember, we should make positive choices, even when we feel negative. Our goal is to drive the pain from their spirit bubbles and replace it with joy. Easy? Not at all! In fact, it's very hard to do because they often fight against us. Worth the effort? Most definitely!

Life experiences must be experienced

I try to make fun of the trauma and disappointment I've dealt with. I do my best to use all my experiences to find happiness and joy. I look at what happened and see what I've learned, even when all seems gloom and doom. I know it may take time, but it does show up. Others have told me that listening to my stories has changed them and given them a new view of their own life. This fills my bubble with more joy.

My first memory of pain

My first clear memory of pain was when I was five-years-old. I suffered a green-stick fracture to my left arm. I've no memory of the accident, but my mother tells me I fell off a wall. I remember the wall;

I thought it fun to walk along. There's something about a wall that draws children and they have no choice but to walk on it. This one was about 1,000 feet long 6 inches high at the lowest, rising to four to five feet high. To a five-year-old, four feet high made it a mountain. Every time I walked to the end, I'd be too scared to jump down.

My older brother, Brian, was also too scared. Each time, we'd plead for help from passing adults. Most times, someone would lift us down. In 1961, cars weren't as common as they are today. A couple of mile walk was a short stroll, so there were plenty of adults around. Today, we'd be stuck there. If we couldn't find a helpful adult, we either had to go back to the beginning or jump down. The start wasn't a wonderful choice, as we'd be late for school. Jumping was a scary choice, yet days later, I'd be on the wall again.

In my memory, the wall is somewhere between 10 and 15 feet high. This is because my perceptions, as a little boy, color my memories. It had to be less than five feet tall; adults could reach up and help us down.

Uphill both ways

My trip to primary school also proves it is possible to go uphill both ways. From our house, we traveled down a hill, which is why the wall got higher and higher. The road goes down to the railway line and back up again, to where the school stood on the other side of the valley. So, both to school and back home, I'd go uphill. The bridge brings back wonderful memories of steam trains. When a train pulled out of the nearby station, there would be a huge amount of steam and all we could see was the smoke. I loved standing there, as the world turned white for a minute or so. Today, the steam trains and the railway line are long gone, as is the bridge with wooden slats and the road has been redesigned completely. My spirit bubble fills to overflowing recalling the memory of the steam and the sound of the train whistle. My amygdala is tickled and I feel wonderful.

This day, I mustn't have been able to find an adult to help me down and I'd jumped, somehow breaking my arm. I was accident-prone, constantly falling, to the point my dad would accuse me of tripping over imaginary matchsticks. I finished off in ER, where they put my arm in a cast. All I remember is the plaster cast being prepared and put on my arm, the horrible itching, and that it caused me a problem with a schoolteacher.

Miss Drysdale

My second-grade teacher, Miss Drysdale, was an older woman. To me, at five, she seemed ancient and stern. She'd become a teacher when female teachers couldn't marry and so had stayed single and childless.

One day, Brian and I were returning to school from lunch through the park next to the school, when in the distance, we saw Miss Drysdale. We decided to shout at her and call her names from behind a small hill. She wouldn't be able to see us and we wouldn't get into trouble, or so we thought. As soon as we got back to school, we were called to the Headmasters office and accused of being rude to Miss Drysdale. I tried to deny it. Unfortunately, Miss Drysdale had seen my cast and realized who the rude boys were.

Although the cast had proven I was the naughty boy; it saved me from the Headmasters favorite punishment, which involved a stick and your hand. We had to hold our hand out in front of us at a specific level. If he didn't think your hand was in the right position, he'd use the cane to move it. Once he was satisfied your quaking hand was in the correct position and, after a pause to maximize the horror, he'd raise the cane high in the air and hit your hand as hard as he could. My broken arm tempered his sadism.

Without the cast, I may have gotten away with it. The headmaster and his sadism is why we didn't want to go back to the start of the wall. Being late, was one of the many petty rules for an automatic caning. Being rude and unpleasant, in the way Brian and I were to Miss Drysdale, should be at the top of the list. The headmaster also decided not to use the cane on my backside, which was his other place of punishment. He'd hit us with the cane, or with a table tennis paddle. He was a sadist who enjoyed punishing boys, not the girls.

If a teacher sent you out of class for being rowdy, we tried to squeeze against the wall, so he couldn't see us. This would result in a caning, unless we were lucky enough to have a girl sent with us. He wasn't being sympathetic or empathetic; he thought beating girls would get him into trouble.

Not Again!

A day or so after the cast came off, I managed to fall over the fireplace in our front room. There was a raised tiled area with a front tile of 3 inches, which I tripped over and fell on my left arm.

I can still recall the bus trip to the hospital, praying I didn't need another cast, as the itching had driven me mad. My hopes and prayers were dashed and I spent another six weeks with a new cast on. My mother introduced me to the beneficial use you can put a knitting needle to. As I'd broken my left arm and I'm right-handed, I still had to go to school and continue being a scoundrel.

They know who I am

I did learn a lesson about not being rude and the fact that, often, "they" do know who we are. For many years, I have found I can't go anywhere without finding people I know, or who know of me. They are friends of friends, or family members, or someone who works with one of my siblings. My family is spread out over the world. Ann and I live in the USA, one sibling hasn't married and lives with my mother; one lives in Switzerland; one in New Zealand and one in England, 220 miles from my mother's house. Somehow, anywhere we go, someone knows me.

My mother goes places and is asked if she is my mother. This irritates her and she'd tell them I'm her son. This still happened after we moved to the USA.

It happens with other people on our behalf. Not too long ago, one of Ann's friends, Sue, was at a visitor's center in St. George, Utah, 400 miles from where we lived in Willard, Utah. A guide asked her where she was from and, when she told them, the guide said she knew someone from Willard, an Andrew Gray, when she was at college. Sue told her he was the daughter of her friend. Even weirder, a family from England was visiting St. George and asked, "The Grays? David and Ann Gray from Newcastle? We know them."

This happens all the time and it started when I decided to call my 2nd grade teacher rude names, while wearing a cast on my broken left arm.

Fighting Pain Finding Joy

Doors are always opening

A happy person isn't a person in a certain set of circumstances, but rather a person with a certain set of attitudes. (Broadcaster Hugh Downs.)

One common idea about life, is that when one door closes, another opens. The idea is we are moving forward through these doors. Some of us spend too much time worrying about the closed one behind us and don't see the door in front. When this happens, we stop moving forward. We may have to worry if the doors are like the ones on the car I owned in 1980. It had acquired the habit of opening the passenger door when someone closed the driver's door. It once did it while I was driving at 75mph and scared the person sitting in the passenger seat. I had to resort to tying the door shut using the seat belt.

The doors I am referring to aren't physical doors, but many of us seem to be trying to fasten the newly opened door shut so we don't have to face what is on the other side.

One of the worst experiences Ann and I went through, involved a door slamming in our faces. The memory brings pain whenever we think about it. I have to work hard to keep the negative emotions it brings from my spirit bubble.

Two-year-old Mandie and six-month-old Marcela left in such a way, the trauma is fresh in our minds years later. They'd come to us, because their mother's drug dealing activities had resulted in her arrest. In this sort of situation, if there's no other family member at home or, the other family members are unsuitable or dangerous to place the child there, CPS will place the child in a foster home.

In Utah, they go to The Christmas Box House temporary children's home, partially funded from the sales of Richard Paul Evan's book of the same name. Workers assess their needs, before they move to a permanent foster home. When there are no places at the Christmas Box House, or they're under the age of two, they go to shelter foster homes. In Texas and most other US states, the children go straight to a foster home.

This involves a placement worker checking a list of licensed homes known to have space, and calling them up. These calls often occurred in the middle of the night. For a change, this one came in the middle of the day. They told us what they knew about the children, which, as always, wasn't much. The only thing they did know which strangely wasn't always correct, was the color of the children's skin.

Hello Mom!

Mandie walked through our back door with a social worker and shouted a cheery "Hello Mom" to Ann. Six-month-old Marcela had withdrawal problems, caused by his intrauterine exposure to drugs and his mother's continuous drug use, since he was born. This made him scream loudly and often, with a neurological scream. The drugs made his brain unable to process all the information coming in and his brain screamed. This is probably an inadequate diagnosis, but ask those who have heard a neurological scream and he or she will use the same sort of definition as I have.

Despite this, we quickly grew to love them both. As their mother wasn't doing the court-mandated services, we expected to have them in our lives for some time. We didn't expect to keep them permanently, but thought we'd have them at least through the end of the year.

Christmas was soon and we bought them presents. Amy, our youngest biological child, was fourteen and we were all excited for the childlike wonder, only a two-year-old has at Christmas. Mandie was incredibly cute and talked up a storm. For a two-year-old, she had a good vocabulary.

Branson, Missouri

We took the children with us on vacation to Branson, Missouri for Thanksgiving and we all enjoyed ourselves immensely. They'd only taken two months to fit into our family. When we took them to a restaurant and shared a table with two policemen, the children stared worriedly at them the whole time. During their removal from home, a policewoman had had to sit on their mother, to put handcuffs on her. Not surprisingly, this traumatized the children. We told the officers why and they spent the rest of the meal proving they were normal people, who had no intention of harming them in any way. The children were impressed and happy to be around them. The policemen impressed Ann and me even more, by paying for our meal.

By the week of Christmas, both children had settled in and we all looked forward to the arrival of Santa. Our older children didn't quite fight over who got to hold Marcela; Mandie loved hugs as well. We've many pictures of them with either Andrew or Amy.

No Santa this year

We'd only been fostering in Texas for five months and were still trying to work out how things worked in another country. We didn't know our rights as foster parents. We received a phone call at 7am on December 22, telling us to bring the children straight down to the CPS office, forty miles away. When I asked why, I was tersely told the judge was sending them home.

The social worker had failed to file some paperwork, from a recent court hearing and the court reluctantly returned the children to their mother's custody. If that happened now, we may well argue the point and leave the worker to deal with any wrath from the court.

We tearfully packed their bags and their six or so sacks of Christmas toys into our car and headed to the CPS office. We took them up to the floor where the social worker was waiting and we handed them over.

Social work is an extremely challenging job. We've worked with some wonderful people, who had the children's welfare as their prime motivator. Social worker pay is inadequate for what they do and, in most places, there are too few workers and far too many children who need their help. Most of the ones we have worked with, have done all

137

they possibly can to reunite families and make the children's experience with the foster care system as pleasant as possible, given what has happened to them. Occasionally, social workers are beaten down from the horror of a job asking too much from them. They almost literally burn out. This is especially true of the ones who are the nicest.

Why so unpleasant?

Marcela and Mandie's social worker wasn't one of those. She most definitely was a zounderkite who couldn't care less about the feelings of some revolting little brats, or the irritating foster parents who, for some reason, seemed to care for the little monsters. She made no effort to make the transition easy, or pleasant. Instead, she seemed to revel in making the handover as hard as possible. A few social workers seem to have no conscience and treat the children as if they were objects without any feelings. She held tightly onto the children, who were by now both crying and screaming loudly as they watched us walk away. We turned a corner and pressed the elevator button with the frightened sound of "mommy, daddy" echoing in our ears.

Goodbyes make for a bad Christmas

This wasn't a good Christmas present for any of us. We haven't seen or heard from them since. Amazed to get her children back, mother did what, to her, was the best idea. She moved away, so CPS could no longer interfere in her life. They were our 17th and 18th foster children. We'd said goodbye to the other 16 children before they arrived and to number 19 two weeks before. Number 20 left the next day. Their goodbye was the hardest we have had. Our spirit bubbles were full of sadness when we said goodbye, so were the children's.

Saying goodbye is part of the process of foster parenting, a cost, if you will. Something that causes an immense amount of pain. The reason many people quit fostering so quickly is the pain it causes. We force ourselves to be positive anyway and then suffer the cruel comments from others about being hardhearted. "**I** could **never** be a foster parent because **I could never** give them up" is a common statement we hear from "friends".

The whole purpose of the foster care system is to offer a stable and safe home for children, for varying amounts of time. How long, is one of the many things over which we have no control, except how we respond to the pain and horror. The loss can quickly negativize our spirit bubbles, driving all joy out.

Had we decided the cruel and callous way we were treated, meant we no longer fostered, we would have no adopted children. Our first adopted child was our 30th foster child and our sixth was # 115. Had we stopped we would never have adopted children 6 through 9 and our life would be totally different from what it is.

One door closes another opens.

Before we left the CPS building, we decided to visit with our own social worker, who had an office a couple of floors below the one where we'd left Mandie and Marcela. She commiserated with us and explained some of what had happened. She then told us about a baby, recently born in Dallas Children's hospital, on the other side of the highway. She could tell us little; except she'd been born with a cleft lip and palette. She also said police were heading to the family home, to remove her sister. If we'd take them, they'd bring her to us.

We drove to the hospital and they took us into the room where the baby was in an incubator. Her mother's drug abuse had removed the baby's choice of being born without physical problems. As her body grew, the drugs, passing through the uterine wall, affected her body. Several problems, including genetics, can cause cleft palate. A person with a cleft palate is more likely to give birth to a baby with one. The likelihood rises from 1 in 700 to 1 in 14. A common cause seems to be the mother's exposure to toxic compounds. These include anticonvulsant drugs; alcohol; cigarette use; nitrate compounds; organic solvents; parental exposure to lead; and illegal drugs (cocaine, crack cocaine, heroin, etc.). Sandy's mother used cocaine.

When our social worker asked us to go to the hospital, we had a choice. We could have said no. We could have said no when we saw the baby. She looked strange, as she had no upper lip or nostrils. There was a hole in the roof of her mouth. We had to learn how to super glue an attachment onto the edge of where her upper lips and nostrils should have been. Without the appliance, eating was impossible, even using a special bottle with an extended nipple that went past the hole in her palette. We also learned how to remove the appliance and clean her mouth.

A social worker's incompetence caused us to lose Mandie and Marcela, and now, we had a newborn baby, who needed our help. We had to learn all the complexities of making it possible for her to eat, but these took us a relatively brief time. More importantly, we had the chance, a method of fighting the pain of losing Mandie and Marcella by finding joy in becoming parents to another needy set of children.

There is a song called Pick Yourself Up. It was written in 1936 by Dorothy Fields with Jerome Kerr composing the music. It has been sung by many people. The chorus says

> *Pick yourself up,*
> *Take a deep breath,*
> *Dust yourself off*
> *And start all over again.*

This is what we did. Things are going to go wrong and cause us pain; it's up to us to pick ourselves up and start over again when they do. It happens to us all at some point.

Who are they and where's my momma and sister?

Sandy's eighteen-month-old sister Bethany also had no choices that Christmas. She was excited to be getting a new sister, but some strange people came and took her to another house, with more strange people. They were the wrong color and spoke funny. She and her family are black; we're white. They also had an odd-looking baby, who they kept saying was her new sister. Her Christmas was full of strangeness.

For us, spiritual, mental and emotional pain had driven all positiveness, all joy out of our spirit bubbles, that morning. We had felt inspired to go see our worker, Toni, to have her make us feel better, with no idea of how. Thankfully, she did and Christmas was saved for us.

Sandy and Bethany's father had a heart wrenching decision to make. Until the investigation was complete and mother had completed all the court-mandated services, including three months of clean urinalysis drug tests, she couldn't live in the same house as her children. He made the incredibly hard choice and asked his wife to leave. He claimed he was unaware of her drug use, as she only used when he was at work.

He was a huge guy with large hands and thick fingers. It was remarkable to watch him concentrate on gluing the appliance to his daughter's mouth and feed her. We used super-glue and, if we got it wrong, we were stuck, and had to hope we had acetone close by.

Dad's life changed, because of his wife's choices. He did what was necessary and made choices, so his daughters could come home. He missed Christmas with both, while background checks made sure it was safe for him to bring them home. I'm sure his bubble was filled with animosity and possibly hatred towards his wife that year, something he has hopefully resolved.

Our role

Ann and my role was to care for his children and there was a lot to do. On Christmas Eve, Ann had to spend 8 hours with Bethany at Children's Hospital, because she had a fever of 103 degrees. A huge issue with fostering is that, even though the State offers Medicaid coverage for all children in care, few doctors choose to take patients who only have Medicaid coverage. Where we lived in Texas, there was one doctor in a 10,000-square mile area.

North of us, the nearest doctor who accepted Medicaid was 100 miles away, east and west were the same. There was one in our local town and then 40 miles south to the next one. If shut, as they were on Christmas Eve, we had to take the children to the only other place available, the emergency room of Children's Hospital in Dallas.

We began teaching Sandy how to eat. It was initially hard for both her and us as was attaching the appliance to make it possible; we learned quickly. Cleft lips and palettes are an easier plastic surgery "fix" and by the age of three, you wouldn't know they ever had the problem.

Saying goodbye to Sandy and Bethany was a success story. Hard on us, as we were losing two more babies, but a success because of where they went. In four weeks, Mother hadn't had the chance to prove she was drug clean and had a long way left to go. Father, however, had the full support of his mother and his extended family and was willing to do what was necessary, to give the loving safety he had thought his wife was providing.

We took the effort to fill their spirit bubbles with love, happiness and joy. We hope they can keep them positively charged. This is why we are foster parents. We look to help children with fighting pain finding joy so they can learn how to positively charge their spirit bubbles. They come with negatively charged ones and leave having had them filled with love and happiness. This helps us forget our pain and fills our spirit bubbles with positivity.

Without even knowing how, we helped them update their plan of happiness. They now have the memory of what **they** did to get this love and happiness. They can use this memory in the future. They also remember being loved and can remember how that felt as well.

Choose wisely

To go back to the door analogy, there are often multiple open doors, or as in our trip across the desert at Dead Horse Point, multiple possible roads, only one of which is the correct one. When we realize we've chosen the wrong one, and head back to where we chose poorly, we're learning.

Sandy and Bethany's mother made some poor choices, forcing her husband to make a horrible choice; his wife or his children. What a decision to have to make! Especially at Christmas. He chose his daughters and presumably hoped his wife got her life sorted out. I don't know if she ever did, as CPS closed the case and we lost touch with the family.

This is life; we make choices and decisions we hope will bring us the most possibility of joy. Some bring temporary pleasure, not necessarily happiness. Long-term joy can bring short-term unhappiness and discomfort. Sandy's dad understood he had a tough decision. He was at a crisis point in his life. Whatever he did, he was at the end of the line.

He had to decide between two horrible choices, his wife, whose selfish choices had forced him into a corner, or his children. He could have whined and complained about how unfair it was to have this crisis thrust on him, and he might have, I don't know.

It Hurts A Lot

Happiness is something you get as a by-product in the process of making something else. (Aldous Huxley)

Mental pain and anguish can be as hard to deal with as physical pain, which of course can cause mental anguish. One discomfort I must deal with started in 1995, when I had the misfortune to contract orchitis. If you're female, this condition is impossible for you to imagine. Orchitis is a swelling of the testicles, a painful condition linked to glandular fever which can make it difficult to have children.

My only concern at the time was I hurt horribly. It felt the same as a hit to the groin, but the pain never went away. If I hadn't been driving, I'd have rolled up in a ball and cried. I was nearly home and I carefully drove the last mile or so. It took me 10 minutes to get out the car and I only moved, because it was beginning to hurt more staying there. I staggered manfully into the house and went to lie on the sofa.

In a macho voice, I asked Ann to contact our doctor, when she had the time. Ann believes I whined, crawled and cried to the sofa. But, who are you going to believe? I waited patiently for him to show up, filling the time by practicing climbing sideways up and down the sofa back, while making small whimpering sounds, similar to the quiet sounds women make during the second stage of labor. After a few millennia, he eventually arrived. He examined the fist-sized swelling at the top of my leg and told Ann to take me straight to ER.

I kept my macho exterior; ignored the pain and walked, head held high, to the car and only had Ann drive because she needed some driving experience. I quickly sat in the passenger sear and we headed to the hospital. Well, that is how I remember it. Ann says I waddled as if I'd lost my horse and, moaning and groaning, staggered slowly to the passenger side and carefully lowered myself to the seat. This took several minutes to do. I do remember waddling into the ER giving a good impression of a man who'd lost his horse. I'm not sure, but the waddling does seem to have enabled me to be quickly triaged and seen by a doctor as soon as we got there.

Stop screaming!

I was put on a gurney, ready for a doctor to torture me. Every time he touched the swollen part, I screamed. He kept telling me to stop screaming and I kept telling him I'd stop screaming, when he stopped poking. The nurse wasn't impressed with my behavior. She also wanted me to stop screaming. To get her message across, she was trying to speak louder than I was screaming. It seems I was causing her mental and emotional pain.

The doctor, having decided I didn't have a strangulated hernia, whatever that was, told the nurse to give me some pain medication. She filled a syringe from a bottle, morphine probably, and told me to turn onto my side. I'd spent the past ten or so minutes, lying on my shoulder blades and ankles, with my back arched and, no other part of my body touching the bed. I slowly and carefully turned onto my side, exposing my naked buttock. Given where I hurt and the part being examined, there was no need to pull my pants, or anything else, out the way. The nurse told me "this will make you forget your pain." Without warning, or swabbing with an antiseptic or anesthetic wipe, she raised the needle above her head and stabbed me, with what I think was gleeful satisfaction.

She was right; I no longer felt the pain in my testicle. After a minute the morphine and the anti-emetic, she'd given me to stop me feeling sick, took effect, and I floated off to my favorite place when hurt, La-La land.

I don't recommend the nurses methods. She received short term joy and happiness to be so unpleasant to me. As far as distraction it worked and the only pain I recall from the evening is that one.

A long trip to the bathroom

I was in hospital for 10 days, connected to a morphine drip on wheels. We traveled everywhere together, very, very slowly. A trip to the bathroom, took most of the morning. If my drip and I took such a trip when dinner arrived, it could become a full-blown civilization before I returned. If you've eaten hospital food, you'll know this isn't necessarily a long time.

I was in a teaching hospital and so was a featured patient for an hour or two each day. My fist-sized lump was poked, prodded, examined and discussed by would-be doctors of both genders. My presence seemed to be optional. Eventually, as there were no complications, I was sent home to finish my recuperation, without my pal the drip, which is I actually missed. It was a joyful day, as I'd enjoyed none of my stay in hospital.

Mononucleosis or Glandular fever seems to cause a recurrence of pain. I know the pain is about to return when the lymph nodes in my mouth grow and hurt. This is my cue to go to the doctors and get some antibiotics. I generally don't need extra pain pills as I already take enough. It's simply another problem to manage. How I manage it, is what matters. As with every problem we deal with in life, we're either a victim, or we're the person who learns how to deal with a problem and turn it from a problem to a learning moment.

Even though I still feel the pain, I find the humor and love to tell the story. One year at a work Christmas Eve party, we somehow got onto the topic of painful experiences. As I told the story of my losing a horse, a workmate ran from the room and upchucked at the idea of what happened to me. He couldn't process the facts without being sick. Telling, or recalling, **this** story makes me laugh and makes my spirit bubble overflow with joy and happiness.

If you want to retell one of your stories, you must be like me and be sure the retelling is not painful to you. If I tell my stories with humor it is cathartic and fills my spirit bubble with joy. If I tell them looking for sympathy, the pain ramps up to 10 out of 10 and my spirit bubble is negatively filled. If retelling your stories is painful to you, you will receive no cathartic release from the retelling, just sadness.

Going on a bear hunt

146

The American folk song, *"Going on a bear hunt"*, has a chorus that talks about obstacles we can't go over, we can't go under and we can't go around. We are left with the choice of going through the obstacle. In the kid's song, the obstacles are fields and rivers.

Our stumbling blocks aren't the same as when hunting bears, but the choices are the same. We can choose what we will do, how can we overcome the obstacle, because we must go through it. There is no option allowing us to stay where we currently are. Stopping in the middle of the road has never been a choice we have. We either choose to make our darkest moment our defining moment or something to learn and grow from.

Leave it

Some experts tell us we should leave the past behind, because it's a country we won't return to. Once something has happened it can't be undone. They are correct, the laws of nature mean we can't turn around, there is no time travel, unless Daniel Smithson from my novel, *There's Always Time*, is real. He finds a way to time travel but still can't change things that have happened.

The experts are also correct about letting go of any negative feelings the trauma brought, being the only way to move forward. Otherwise, we're stuck at that point in the road and unable to progress. Those with us are also stuck at that point. People behind us will finish off jostling, trying to get past, as will anyone coming the other way. If jostling has no effect, they are stuck with us. Only when we choose to move on down the road; can we go any further. The more negative emotions in our spirit bubble, the more likely we'll try to stay where we are. If our plan of happiness is written to ensure victim-hood, a negatively charged spirit bubble and a desire to be stuck in the past reliving an unpleasant event, we would seem to be succeeding. If not, we need either a change of direction or voluntarily move on from where we are. If we don't we will eventually be pushed off the road or down the mountain.

With me, as soon as I get the heavy feeling at the top of my leg, I know I need some antibiotic. I've learned there's no immediate joy, only discomfort, but I'm confident I can manage without having to go find my friend the drip.

I have no choice, because I'm now allergic to morphine and, if I take some, I get hives and itch.

Humor

RSD doesn't mean I can ignore new pain, it means I know how to handle it better than others may do. Or as I used to. I can't go around it, I can't go over it, I can't go under it, and so I must go through it.

My method is to use humor. When humor is absent from our lives for a long time, we're clinically depressed. If this is you, it's essential you visit with your doctor. In many cases, clinical depression can only be resolved with medication. Even then, medication can't solve all the problems. We also need laughter in our lives. Note I say also; I cannot manage at all without taking my medications. They **don't** remove all the pain, not even close. I use laughter as another layer of medication along with my prescription drugs, Laughter makes stress easier to handle. I've found when I laugh, I feel better. Being able to laugh at myself is even better.

As well as being able to laugh at ourselves, being able to laugh at nothing is also helpful. I don't mean literally; you might get locked up in a padded room. I mean laughing when others expect it, but you don't feel there's anything funny.

When life isn't the way we want it to be, we can get depressed. Having to walk as if I've lost my horse is depressing. There's no fun either. I had the right to be depressed, didn't I? Well, yes, I did. Up till then, it was the worst pain I'd ever suffered As there's no positive benefit from being depressed, my spirit bubble was filled with unhappiness and was negatively charged for the whole time I was in hospital. I can choose to remember that feeling and become depressed or I can choose to remember the funny side.

I know that the worse we feel mentally, spirituality, or emotionally, the worse we feel physically. It circles round and the more depressed, the more physical pain we're aware of and the worse we feel mentally, spiritually or emotionally. Laughter helps lift depression. What should we do when life isn't funny? Laugh anyway! When we're depressed, what we otherwise may find funny, we tend to go blah at. Fight the urge and laugh anyway. This makes us feel better and each later laugh gets easier. Happiness shines through our faces whether we smile or not, smiling helps, though. Our positively charged spirit bubble ensures it.

Smile at yourself

A psychologist in a mental institute tried an experiment, where, each time they saw themselves in a mirror, patients had to smile at their reflections. The patients who smiled got better 50% faster. I'm not a mental patient, but I do force myself to smile when I don't particularly find anything is amusing. I always feel better. Laughter makes me feel even better.

A visit to Pocatello, Idaho might help. They take smiling so seriously it's illegal to have any other facial expression. The ordinance was passed by Mayor George Philips in 1948, after a particularly long, dark winter had everybody feeling depressed.

However... There always seems to be a 'however", or a 'but' we must consider. This one is different though, this however says life is only as hard as **we allow** it to be, chronic pain, or not. If we can laugh over what we can't control, even if it is only internally, to ourselves, we **will** feel better.

How am I? I feel awful!

I start each day feeling dreadful. No real sleep and a night full of hurting, leaves me tired and grumpy each morning. When I go to the bathroom and look in the mirror, I know I look bad. I force myself to smile, and make sure the smile radiates into my face and eyes then breathe deeply. The man who looks back at me looks a lot better.

He would still scare you, so I'm doing no selfies.

When I focus on not taking life, and all its challenges, too seriously, by laughing instead of than stressing, I can overcome any hurdle. If there's nothing to laugh about, I remind myself of what I've

149

laughed over in the past. Laughter helps me stay balanced during tough times. I consider my blessings; and use them to help me laugh, by tickling and teasing them.

It would be wonderful if my sleep improved, but nothing seems to do that. Whoops, that's a gripe and, as I cannot allow negative thoughts to fill my spirit bubble, please ignore this paragraph.

I have found that with practice, I can now laugh to order. No matter how much physical, mental, spiritual or emotional pain I am feeling, I can make myself laugh because I want to. This forces positive emotion into my spirit bubble and pushes the negative emotions out.

I don't always succeed in acting as if, especially when others are unwilling to change. This negatives my spirit bubble and it is easy to find negative emotions waiting to get me. I may have to seek forgiveness for losing my temper, even though I'm not in the wrong in the first place. I have to take a very deep breath and do whatever I need to do to **act as if** the other person was **not** horribly unpleasant to me. The concept of trying to **act as if** is the spirit's defense mechanism. It is trying to help us remain strong. I may have to use this defense mechanism a lot or a little, but using it helps **<u>me.</u>**

Trying to get others to understand how it feels to be in constant chronic pain is very difficult, because they have no reference point. They break bones or otherwise hurt themselves, or get hurt. They go to the doctor, get a cast put on or get some antibiotics or whatever is needed for the current trauma. Then they get better and everything is good. It may take a while, but it does get better eventually

My body doesn't work that way anymore. I have a trauma and the pain stays. I go through everything as others, except for that one point, the pain stays. I have to work out how to manage it after I am supposed to have "got better."

Who left that hole lying around?

Happiness can be defined, in part at least, as the fruit of the desire and ability to sacrifice what we want now for what we want eventually.   (Stephen Covey)

My ability to fall over nothing means I've suffered many cuts and scrapes, and several sprains, as well as broken bones. In fact, I fell off the arm-smashing wall again, this time spraining my ankle. I hobbled home in tears, received a lecture on walking on the wall and told to hobble off to school. My tears and showing how much I hurt did me no good and I hobbled off, as best I could. I managed to get back before the headmaster and had no problems over a potential caning.

The hidden hole

11 years had passed before I decided to break another bone. I got my first motor bike when I was 16, a yellow Honda C70. A 70cc scooter type bike with three crash gears and a top speed of 40mph on the flat, 20 to 30 mph uphill and occasionally, 50mph down a steep hill, with a strong wind behind you.

The motor bike was faster than a bicycle and took no effort, but getting anywhere still took a long time. A good example is when Brian and I took a 300-mile trip, back to visit old friends, on our motor bikes. His bike was a Honda 50, with even lower speed abilities. The trip took us 2 days and we had to camp overnight, at the halfway point. Mother Nature decided we weren't suffering enough, taking a small eternity to get anywhere, so had a rainstorm drench our tent. We woke up soaking wet. At least the sun and the air helped us dry, and for the first couple of hours, we steamed.

I am happy remembering it. I don't dredge up anything but the silliness of steaming along at 30mph.

151

Oh look! A pothole

One Saturday, around Christmas 1971, I was heading home on my super-powerful motorbike, when I found a large pothole someone had carelessly left in the middle of the road. Instead of being sensible and driving around this entrance to the nether world, the bike's front wheel decided to go deep into the hole. The careless part was, it was hidden around a corner. I decided this would be a suitable time to practice the sort of flying I'd tried as a child. I was no more successful and, as soon as I flew over the handlebars, gravity noticed and sent me smacking into the ground. I did what I thought was a graceful roll and got straight back up. I knew there was a large gravel truck behind me and I needed to get out of its way. I'd failed at flying and didn't want to see how well I'd do, if we tried to argue with the truck.

The Washington Post has an annual contest where readers have to come up with alternative meanings for words. Flatulence was redefined as an emergency vehicle that transports victims of steamroller accidents. Behind me was a gravel truck, not a steamroller, but I believed if I didn't move, I'd need a flatulence. As I grabbed the handlebars, my right shoulder complained loudly and I dropped the bike. The truck easily managed to stop. The low speed ability of my motor bike probably saved me from more injuries.

Back to hospital we go.

Someone called the police and I was whisked off to hospital in an ambulance. The second of several trips I've made in an ambulance. The first was when I was 18 months old and decided drinking engine oil was a great idea. My father was changing the oil in his motor bike and used one of my old cups. A poor choice for us both. I finished off in an ambulance and then in an oxygen tent at the hospital. My dad lost his job when his boss, the head nurse or matron, at the same hospital, was upset my dad didn't let them know he wouldn't be into work that night. My dad suggested the matron had a lower endoscopy. He worked as a bus conductor for a few months, until swallowing his pride and apologizing. He never said how that meeting went; I do know that for the rest of his working life, he worked in the nursing profession, so it must have gone well. I believe this choice was a much better one than staying as a bus conductor.

I caused a traffic jam

One trip I laugh about was when I broke my neck in a car accident, in 1992. I went to the hospital on the city's eastern edge and they decided I needed transporting to the one on the western side. At rush hour! I made the journey sandbagged and strapped securely in an ambulance that crossed through the city center at 5 mph, with its lights and sirens on, following an equally slow moving police car. I believe there are people still stuck in that traffic jam.

At the hospital after the 1971 motorbike accident, they x-rayed my arm and shoulder and told me I'd broken my clavicle, the medical term for our collarbone. My father arrived at the hospital a short while later and took me home. I don't know who kindly retrieved my super bike, but it also made its way home. Later the next day, I realized I had banged my head, when I fainted from a concussion. Up to then, I believed it silly to be told to watch the "patient" for 24 hours, but I proved myself wrong when all the blood drained out of my face and I hit the ground, without causing myself any further injury, thankfully.

Looked after by a girl, no less

A few days later, my father and I traveled from London to Newcastle to stay with friends, who still lived in the village we'd moved from a few years earlier. This was the same journey Brian and I had taken two days to make. A motor car instead of a slow motor bike means the journey only took 5 hours.

We were visiting my first crush, Yvonne's, family. Not only did I get to sleep in her bed, while she shared with her sister, she became my personal nurse. My right arm was in a sling with my hand fastened to my left shoulder, so I couldn't move my collarbone. It hurt to try.

Yvonne helped me with what I'd normally use my right arm and hand for. She even tucked me into bed, as it was against the wall and I had difficulty shuffling into the space. As the accident had only occurred a few days earlier, and I'd recently recovered from the concussion, I'd not worked out how to eat left-handed, so she helped me with that too. At the time, it made the pain bearable. Without the broken bone, she'd probably have ignored me.

With my right hand stuck against my left shoulder, I couldn't write and, this time, I missed school for a while. Eventually, the doctors removed the sling, allowing me to use my right hand and I returned to school a few weeks after Christmas vacation. I couldn't ride my motorbike, as that needed two hands and the collarbone still hurt. I had to learn how to walk to school again, this time up a steep hill, but only from home to school. At home, there was no girl willing to help me, as my sister didn't think I was incapacitated. My baby sister may have helped me, but she was only a few months old, her part was limited to not having big brother cuddle her all the time.

Officially a biker, now

People told me, because I'd broken a bone while riding a motorcycle, I was now an official biker, even if I had such a slow machine. A couple of months later, I bought my first real motor bike, the sort where you straddled the gas tank which was in front. It was a Honda CB 175 with twin carburetors and a powerful engine, despite the relatively small engine size.

I often drove at speeds of up to 100 mph. To reach this speed, I had to lie horizontally with my chin resting on the gas tank and my feet over the flasher stalks on either side, at the back. My hands were on the steering column, working the accelerator and front brake. This cut out all wind resistance and added 20 mph. When I needed to slow down, change gears, or stop, I sat sit up quickly. None of the accidents I had on that bike, were to do with speed.

Oil Leak

I had a cartoon-like accident when I was following an oil truck, which was leaking oil, causing me to lose control of the bike. I was doing about 45 mph, so laying it down was no easy choice. I was wearing my full leather gear and the road was slick with oil. I quickly sat up, but didn't slow down. There I am, sliding at 45 mph, with my bike sliding next to me. Fortunately, there was no other traffic and nothing for me to hit and when my bike and I stopped sliding, I simply got up and continued. I didn't think of calling the police and suing the tanker owner for the harm I suffered. Even today, I can't see any purpose in doing so, as I came to no harm. I remember it all with joy, which is more important.

Circus

Talking of my leathers, a policeman, who'd watched one of my crazy stunts, stopped me. I'd reached behind me to the box on the back of my bike, lifted the lid, retrieved my leather driving gauntlets, closed the lid and put them on, all the time keeping control as I drove the bike at 30mph. He asked to see my license and after I gave him my documents, he told me he didn't want to see that license; he wanted to see my circus performer license. I said I didn't have one and he told me not to drive around town performing circus tricks, without a license. His good humor saved me from a couple of tickets and he let me go with a friendly warning.

The traffic police have stopped me since, but he was the friendliest and the wackiest. I'm not a crazy or dangerous driver; I have simply driven an average of 100,000 miles each year and accidents and police stops seem to occur at specific intervals. Insurance company data show accidents occur every 70,000 miles. I've managed to be in a car accident approximately every 5 years.

Doing the speed limit

I've been stopped a few times for driving exactly the speed limit late at night. This is apparently how a drunk driver tries to avoid detection. I'd notice a cop car behind me and leave the car on cruise control. A half-mile or so later, the blue lights would come on and I'd stop.

The police officer would notice the lack of alcohol on my breath and I'd talk pleasantly to him or her. We'd chat for a while then leave.

I have learned that positive communication works. I have occasionally received traffic tickets.

Even pleasantness hasn't stopped me from getting one.

My spirit follows my plan of happiness, which says to try to be pleasant and friendly, to everyone I speak to. Unfortunately, I fail, but I'm going to keep on trying. I've no intention of quitting and becoming a grumpy old man.

When we are in any type of pain, especially the type of emotional pain stress causes, the chances are we'll find everything annoying and are likely to shout. This sort of communication succeeds wonderfully, often at 100%. Unfortunately, what it succeeds in is filling the spirit bubbles of all around us with negativeness.

Even the most positive person with a spirit bubble overflowing with joy, somehow finds it hard not to respond in kind to a person shouting at them. I force myself to take a deep breath and use the thalamic cortical pause when I find myself shouting. It is possible to say the same thing with an angry voice and a cheerful voice and be understood differently. Even "I love you" sounds unbelievable with an angry voice. I have tried it many times with babies when I have said nasty words with a loving, kind voice and had them giggle because they don't know what it means to be a smelly, nasty, scum-bag, but they recognize the loving tone it is said in. My goal, to fill my spirit bubble and all those I meet with joy, needs me to use a cheerful voice. How successful am I? We'll call it a work in progress. Each time I fail, I start again.

Please don't shout

I know how hard it is to be on both sides of this communication issue. All I can offer is suggestions. The hardest part of this is that I know "all the answers" but I don't always like or appreciate them. I know I shouldn't shout, yet I still have a problem with doing it. I shout a huge amount less than I used to. My children can attest to the fact that it is possible to push Dad to a point where he shouts. Naturally, these are the only times they remember and will claim I shout at them all the time. I have to control my response so that I don't allow my spirit bubble to fill with negativity.

If we are the person doing the shouting, we should accept the request from the other person and do everything in our power to calm ourselves. Take a deep breath, count to 10 and force a smile and quietly repeat what we screeched, this time in a calm and controlled voice. We should also smile if we can.

If we are on the receiving end, but responded in kind, do the same thing, but go to the person and apologize for shouting. Shouting at someone for shouting is the most insane communication there is. We should ask if there is anything we can do to help with whatever they are stressed about. They may say no, but they will probably remember our offer.

But I'm not shouting

One issue about shouting I deal with is whether I am shouting, or simply raising my voice. I know how to project my voice so that I can be heard in a large crowded room, even without a microphone.

I have a naturally loud voice. I can still be heard, when I believe I am speaking quieter than if I whispered. It's important we check the body language of others we believe are angry. My children have learned the importance of checking my eyes before worrying about the volume of my voice. If my eyes aren't angry, I'm not angry. If someone is angry, their body language will show anger. If they are stressed, their body language will show it.

Good Communication

Effective communication seems to begin early in life. Kalyn proved to us that little ones can communicate with other babies, even though they can't talk..

This, though, wasn't talking; it was total communication with no speech. Kalyn was nine months old, two months older than Matthew, who could get around in a commando crawl, but not "proper" crawling on his hands and knees. We had wood floors, so he had no problem commando crawling. Kalyn did and decided she'd teach him how to crawl properly. She crawled over, went head-to-head with him for a few minutes and then crawled off, turning around to see if he was following. She tried this for a few minutes, and decided to try a different method. She crawled next to him, went head-to-head again until he pushed himself up on his hands and knees. Once she was satisfied, she crawled off, again showing him how. He was still unable to do anything more than rock backwards and forwards. She tried for several more minutes, before giving up on him. He did eventually learn to crawl, but not that afternoon. The communication between them was amazing to watch. We don't know at what level they were speaking, but they **were** communicating.

This is the sort of communication needed to handle all types of pain. Instead of two little children under the age of one, it's our spirit and our body. Occasionally, especially with teenagers, it would be nice to be able to communicate that way. I may have been able to overcome the standard teenage answer of "I don't know!" to every question. In my house, because shouting is a teenager's normal response to anything, as they're stressed from being a teenager, we get a lot of practice trying to not shout back.

Pain Gates

Give yourself up to this moment. Dare to see it. Now look down at your feet; slip out of those invisible tethers. Then ask: Where would you take yourself right this moment if you walked toward your most heartfelt dream? What would your life look like? What would your body look and feel like? What level of energy would you have? What might be your favorite activity? What would your daily life include? Imagine happiness – the sweet glow of inner contentment, the way it tastes, smells, and feels.
(Chris Downie)

The hurt part of our body and our brain are in close communication while that part hurts. Unless you suffer with the condition where you don't feel pain, you will find this communication occurring every day.

For me, with RSD, this means there is constant communication between the brain's pain gates and most of my body. The messed up sympathetic nervous system is constantly trying to fix the physical trauma, which is no longer occurring. To gain some peace from the pain caused by the vasoconstriction and other nerve processes occurring in the damaged parts, I need to interrupt those messages.

Simplistically put, pain is received through gates. I say simplistically, because I want no hassle from brain experts, who will tell me there is a lot more to it than this. I agree, but this **is** what happens. The pain message pushes through the gates and the limbic system processes it. The gates have powerful springs, which slam shut and lock, until the current pain is processed.

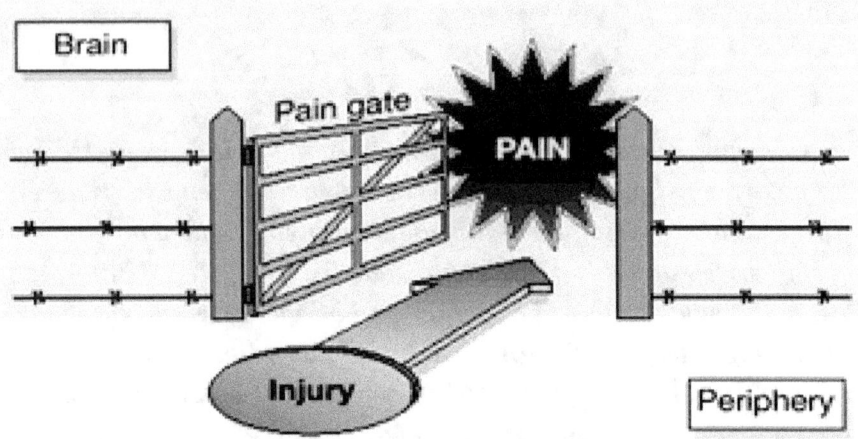

We learn how to process pain as we grow. We write programs to process all pain and automatically run them as needed. We may not know how rubbing the part of our body we banged stops it hurting, yet we know it works. What happens, again simplistically put, is the messages from the rubbing get to the pain gates faster than the original bang. The gates are busy processing the discomfort from us rubbing the spot. This is a small pain and, the protocol most of us has in place is to ignore it. When the slower pain from the original bang arrives, micro seconds later, it's ignored because the gate is shut.

The best example of this is when we prove why we have shins and bang it on a chair. Vigorously stroking the shin minimizes the soreness, at least until we use it to find another piece of furniture.

Closing the gates

I've learned how to close the pain gates and make the pain go down without rubbing. This is important, because, the part of me hurting will hurt even more when touched. My left arm, where the RSD began, is the worst at this. The wind blowing on my bare arm feels as if someone is firing red-hot needles at me. Merely touching the arm often feels as if I've been thumped or rough sandpaper is being rubbed over my arm. This means I must find a different method to lower the discomfort. I confuse people by backing away, if they appear to be about to slap me on my arm.

Those who know me apologize because they know this, but have forgotten.

When my entire body hurts, as happens a lot, I can't rub the affected part. I feel like the person who had being knocked unconscious in an accident. When she wakes, she begins to check her body to see what's broken and is horrified to find everything she touches hurts horribly. Only after a few minutes, during which her brain begins to process what has happened, does she realize the "only" damage is a broken hand. I'd be ecstatic if this was true for me, but it isn't and... see how rapidly and easily I can call a pity party?

GATE CLOSING! GATE CLOSING!

I lower the pain levels by picturing the pain gates in my mind. I imagine a large steel shutter and, closing my eyes, bring the shutter down in front of the pain gates. At the same time, I breathe slowly and deeply and do what I refer to as the DC Comics ®Clark Kent / Superman transformation. I stick my chest out, shoulders back and stomach in. I straighten my back and push upwards.

As the pain levels drop, I relax my face muscles, my shoulders and arms. The pain goes away and stays away, as long as the shutters are down. Unfortunately, this takes effort and is where I often need the help of others to find the strength.

Validation

One of the hardest and most important choices I must make is to select who to validate with. Getting this wrong can be catastrophic, as I've personally found out. Some people not only don't care, they're willing to go as far as to call the police on us.

The reason it can be catastrophic has to do with our perception of complaining. The synonyms for the word complaining include bad-tempered, irritable, argumentative, belligerent, cranky, disagreeable, tetchy, grouch and grumpy. Instead of 7 dwarves, here are 9 crabs permanently in a bad mood.

I have a relative who often fit these definitions.

161

If she ordered a cup of coffee, she'd find a problem, every time. Too hot, too cold, too many little cups of cream, too few cups of cream, the waitress slammed the cup down or put it 3 inches too far away. I'm sure you know someone like this. They are complaining to get sympathy, except, when we offer a solution, they will argue our solutions are no good. Their foot hurts, so we suggest several good doctors we've dealt with. For whatever reason, they find there is an issue with them all. They shoot down every suggestion we make. If we don't offer help, they complain we didn't, because we don't care.

These people may be top complainers, but we all complain at times. Complaining can serve a good purpose. The coffee may well be cold, so send it back and get a new one. If we don't complain, nothing changes. Complaining for the sake of it, is a pointless waste of time.

I don't need a solution

Validation **is** complaining, but it's asking for support and confirmation, **not a solution**. Many times, we may well be grumbling, but we aren't looking for a solution. With validation, all we want is agreement from another person that we do have the right to be upset; that we're justified in thinking life is sucky at this specific moment in time.

Emotional validation is a form of communication where we learn about, understand, and express acceptance of another person's emotional experience. We're acknowledging that what happened is real, logical and understandable. There's no need to even agree or approve. Validation is nonjudgmental and, especially when dealing with someone with chronic pain, it involves eye contact, nodding and showing we're listening,

Emotional validation is the opposite of emotional invalidation, in which the other person's emotional experiences are rejected,

I need to validate often. My problems aren't solvable. What I need is the ability to vent, to blow off steam and that is it. What I don't want, or need, is someone telling me how I'm mistaken. Unless …

There are times when we may well be mistaken and part of validating can involve helping us see things differently.

It's easy to think of life as if we are heading down the mountain, across the desert to our destination. We have little idea where we are heading and what's up ahead. We can convince ourselves that life will be better when we get married or after we are married, we have a child, or another. We're upset when we find our children are too young and we expect our lives will be better when they're older. But they are teenagers now and …. Well, teenagers!

We tell ourselves life will be better when the house is paid off, we get a better job, a nicer car, when the children get married, when we retire. Then we die and life was not what we wanted it to be.

Life is a journey with obstacles and the obstacles make us grow. Bills constantly come due and there's always something to do. As we learn how to overcome the obstacles, the next one seems to be easier to deal with. Enjoy life now, find happiness wherever we can, even when dealing with major obstacles and challenges.

Now is the time to find joy. Anything else makes us a victim.

Celiac's Disease

I received a phone call at about 7pm on December 23rd, 2012, telling me the results of the dozens of tests I'd recently had, including 39 vials of blood. I have Celiac's disease. How to ruin a person's Christmas! Nearly all the food I enjoy eating is now "dangerous" to me. Most of what I can eat, I don't like anyway and the substitutes for what I did enjoy, taste the same as I imagine cardboard does.

After 6-months on a gluten-free diet I can no longer eat "normal" food and when I say there's nothing to eat, or that I want to eat, I don't need to hear gluten free food has come a long way. If there's no gluten-free food available to me right now, there is nothing to eat. I don't want to spend time cooking; I want a snack, now! The pantry, fridge and freezer may well be filled to overflowing with food, but it all contains gluten!

What I need from others is acceptance that I'm unhappy with the current state of affairs and have the right to feel hard done to, **at this moment**. I'll be fine in a few minutes. Right now I'm unhappy. I don't need or want someone to argue I'm wrong, judge me, or tell me there are children starving in Africa. I never understood how me eating my Brussels sprouts, would stop a child in Africa being hungry. The other one of those comments I find hard to swallow is the one that says something like my calf was hurting from running up the hill; then I saw a man with only one leg running past me. How does that help with the pain in my calf? Has the pain gone away now that I have seen a man with a prosthetic leg run past? The answer is no! I'd like to be validated that I have the right to have a sore calf and that's it.

My favorite pain management method is talking. I never pass the opportunity to talk to people. I talk to sad looking strangers and try to make them cheer up; this makes me more cheerful. As I pass, I tell them to smile. This surprises them, but they smile and I tell them they feel better, don't they? Nearly every time they agree with me. My spirit bubble fills with joy when I try to fill other people's with joy.

Head patting

Even though validation is listening and little more than the occasional, "I'm sorry", few of us are capable, or willing, to offer this service. I'm not too good myself. What might help could be to begin the tirade with the statement, "I'm simply venting, but …" so the other person knows we need validation.

This will hopefully let them know we don't want them to solve the problem or show us where we're going wrong. Hopefully! If not, we may have to be that little more forceful in reminding them.

Until I got RSD, I was unsympathetic when it came to illness. I had to believe someone was ill, before taking loving care of him or her. If there was any hint of "swinging the lead", I was unsympathetic.

Many years ago, my eldest son Simon who has cerebral palsy was complaining of some pain and I suggested the way I'd show him sympathy was to pat him on the back of the head. He took this in the

164

humorous way intended and I patted his head. A few days later, he fell and badly hurt his elbow. I asked if he wanted sympathy and he thought about it for a minute. He believed he should receive sympathy, he felt he needed sympathy and we as his family should offer some. However, history suggested all he'd get was a pat on the back of the head. He nevertheless asked for some sympathy not involving having his head patted. His sister came and cuddled him and I patted him on the back of the head. I've learned I should have hugged him and validated his emotional distress.

It's important when we have a healthy family, to be happy they're healthy, not angry or jealous they are. This isn't easy. Generally, others aren't interested, and possibly don't care, we're worse than they are, when they are ill. This is where **acting as if** becomes essential. We need to act as if **we are** interested in their problems and show we care, even if we think we don't. We get to be actors and it's essential our performance is first-rate. We need to **act as if** a lot of things that are far from being acceptable to us, actually are. This is the only way to fight the pain and find joy.

Self-Validation

If there's no one willing, or able, to validate with, this may be a time for some introspection. I do this a lot, as I occasionally wonder if I'm making it all up. It would be wonderful if morning was the next thing I'm aware of after I fell sleep and it didn't hurt to do things. Then I do practically anything, and realize this is my world. However, I still need to vent, I still need validation. What do I do? What can I do? The answer is to do it myself. I act as if someone else does care, me!

Probably the most important communicating we do, is with ourselves, our self-speak. The art of talking to ourselves for encouragement, either aloud or silently and mentally.

One way to deal with the emotions of being way down and depressed over the slings and arrows of outrageous fortune, as Shakespeare has Hamlet say in his famous "To be or not to be" soliloquy, is to do as I do and make fun of what's happening and distract ourselves. Laughter refills our reservoirs.

We can talk to ourselves about our emotions. I've found it helpful to write in my journal. Using a journal to vent is a simple and powerful way to get rid of some pent-up emotions. It is also never judgmental. I am not going to tell myself how I am wrong feeling the way I currently do. That will not help me. I am writing how I feel at the moment and getting rid of the negative emotions blocking up my spirit bubble.

Being positive

At times, I have to force myself to be positive. I may have to search for something positive, but they are there and writing them down, is even more cathartic as writing the unpleasant ones. Most doctors I've seen, over the last 20 or so years, have mocked me for using the word cathartic. I'm not sure why, as it's a great word. It means "the process of releasing, and thereby providing relief from, strong or repressed emotions." Crying is a cathartic action.

If no one can be helpful, I imagine what I'd want others to say, if they were supportive. I either say it to myself, or write it in my journal. I use an "as if" attitude and act as if life was better. It may take a while to regain control but it does happen.

A close friend had a problem with their spouse continuously finding fault. It took me more than 40 years to realize it was handled with the "as if" method, acting as if the nasty remarks weren't said. I found it amazing how he managed to do this as I was present when many of the nasty things were said. I still need to learn from him.

Low point

Here is a journal entry from the recent past.

I'm at one of the lowest points I've been since the 2002 accident. I'm having another flare up of orchitis and am on antibiotics. I'm suffering an elevated level of pain everywhere and I hurt standing, sitting and lying down. I'm

166

getting even less sleep than normal, and I find it even harder to manage the discomfort.

At the same time, I feel as if everything I do is being second-guessed. Instead of getting gratitude for what I do for others, I'm being told it isn't good enough, that I'm making it up, I'm not suffering at all and should do everything an able-bodied person can do. Someone seems to find fault with everything I say or do.

I write people email, but they don't respond then get angry with me when I ask why. In fact, one person knows a cop and had him come and humiliate, offend and attack me in a belligerent, unpleasant way, because I'd emailed to their work account at 12:30am. He told me this was harassment.

I must deal with an 'automatic no' situation where regardless of the question or the person asking, the answer is an immediate no. Not from me, from others.

Nearly everything that makes life enjoyable has been taken away from me. Food, sleep, sports, walking, running, lying down, sitting and doing anything involving lying down, sitting, walking or running are painful and impossible, I have no super powers, so flying isn't a choice I have.

I still have all the stressors of children with problems caused by mistreatment in the womb by their biological mothers, a wife who gets seriously ill for several days every four to six weeks and trying to keep going myself. I can't handle the emotional effect and I cry a lot. Stress and depression makes pain worse and, there feels as if there is no way out of this downward spiral.

I can't see your reaction, but I know I sound pitiful, so I have to believe you're visualizing me being just as pitiful. For me, then and now, however, it is cathartic. As my life is often this way, re-reading it is as good as writing it down is and makes me feel better.

Healing ourselves

167

The hardest part was letting go of the emotion of being down. In life, there are excuses and reasons. A reason is why I cannot do something; an excuse is why I won't do it.

My son Simon has cerebral palsy. This is both a reason and an excuse. He can't run, but he can walk. If he wants to get from point A to point B quickly, it will take longer for him than an able-bodied person, or he can simply not bother. I am proud to say that he doesn't quit and say he can't do it, even when he falls and hurts himself, he picks himself up, dusts himself down and continues on with what he was doing.

For me, the negative events of that day were both a reason and an excuse. They'd drained all my reservoirs and my batteries were flat. My get up and go, had got up and gone, but I'd no idea where. I had to rise above it all, because no one would do it for me. A person who feels appreciated, is much more likely to do what they must do and I was feeling unappreciated.

I was not necessarily unappreciated, but I sure felt as if I was. There is an enormous difference! This is where and when I needed to use all the tools in my toolbox, all the apps I'd developed. I succeed at pain management because I've learned to control the pain gates. This doesn't work too well with mental, spiritual and emotional pain.

The tool for these pains I use the most, is laughter. I laugh at most everything I can and this relieves the stress. I focus on not taking life, and all its challenges, too seriously, by laughing not stressing, I have found doing this means I can overcome any hurdle. If I can't find anything to laugh about, I remind myself of what I have laughed at in the past. Laughter helps me stay balanced during tough times. I have learned how to act as if what is happening is funny and laugh, even when I want to cry. At times, I have done both together. I can feel dreadful and see one of my grandchildren. I have two choices here; stay down and depressed, or force joy and happiness into my voice and say something nice to them. I pick up the little ones and make sure my face is turned so the pain can't be seen.

A reason is why it is <u>impossible</u> for me to do something right now – I cannot.

An excuse is why I <u>don't want</u> to do something.

I will not.

Validating other's pain

When we're in constant pain, we don't necessarily recognize others can be unwell. At the end of 2014, my family all caught the influenza. One child took it one step further and caught pneumonia. I had two choices, give in or keep going. What I have all the time feels like the flu. Even though I felt worse than normal, I decided to persevere, to stay the course, to carry on. While the others lay around moaning, I did my best to look after them. When they recovered, they were back to normal. I stayed behind and had to grin and bear it. Those are the only choices open to me; quit, or grin and bear it and carry on with life.

I suffer with far more than the flu, every day and night, 24/7 etc.

I get no sympathy, or even acknowledgment I feel worse than they do, so why should I give them sympathy and keep going?

When they're sick, I play nurse, even though I'm also feeling sick. When they're better, I still feel awful, but no one cares, no one is the least bit interested in helping me.

This sounds childish, but it's the reality **if I want to be a victim**, stuck in victim mentality mode. Please note, it's only the reality of a person who **wishes** to be, or remain, a victim. My personal plan of happiness has instructions to stop me falling into victim-hood. This actually **is** my reality, but I can't be a victim, I don't want to be one. I therefore must find a way around it.

My role was to give service to my family because I love them. It is true, at my best I feel worse than they do when they are ill, but I have in some way got used to it and can give help where and when it's needed. I can validate them.

Chocolate!

As well as laughter, I try chocolate. I once saw a tee shirt with the words, "in the beginning was the word." On the back, it read, "And the word was chocolate." There's also the suggestion that on the eighth day, God made chocolate and had He intended us to be thin, he wouldn't have bothered.

Chocolate has a duel effect on me. It makes me feel better mentally, but somehow makes pain worse when I over indulge.

I originally wrote "if" but I realized it is usually "when".

Chocolate also makes me put weight on, at the rate of one pound per piece imagined. Free radicals are thought released. They combine with roaming thingamajigs, and along with the whatchamacallits, add pounds to my body, when I only think about the heavenly stuff. I still want to eat it, though. I agree with Dave Barry, "Your hand and your mouth agreed many years ago that, as far as chocolate is concerned, there is no need to involve your brain."

I've tried all the tricks to avoid this weight gain and I don't mean calorie watching. There are 500 calories in a piece of chocolate, what exercises can I do, to use up those calories? No, I break the chocolate into pieces and put them on a high shelf so the calories will fall out. For some reason this doesn't seem to work, but I'm willing to keep on experimenting. I wonder if freezing the chocolate to make the calories die will be more successful. I'll let you know.

Exercise or exorcise

I didn't try exercise. I have both a reason and an excuse when it comes to exercising. Running hurts, lifting anything more than 5lbs hurts and I have nothing but excuses, with the other types of exercise.

I wonder if we have been making a mistake in the English language. We don't hear much about exorcising today and I wonder if those crafty devils, the ones who once possessed our ancestors, gave up on the demonic-possession route. They took time off in some nicer spot in Hades, there to relax and enjoy the pains of a lost soul as much as is inhumanly possible.

But, what do we hear about? Exercising the fat out of our bodies. Coincidence? I don't think so! People have stopped "exorcising" and begun "exercising" and the devils now possess our rear ends, hips, thighs and bellies. Some of us have much larger devils than others, or perhaps more individual devils. When I binge on Dairy Milk chocolate and ask myself "What possessed me to do that?" I know it's the Chocolate-Beast I've allowed into my body, along with his friends: French Fry, Pop Guzzler, and Cookie Monster. You all know I'm right. I know our children think the Cookie Monster is a cuddly Sesame Street character, but they're wrong!

Our bodies are supposed to be temples, and as the scriptures say, "Let thy temple not be fatty." Wait. That is TV. But, when has television advertising ever led us astray?

Millions of people have added years to their lives by spending a mere two hours a day in the gym. For those of us who are possessed, I apologize. Not so much to you, as to the devils inside you, whom I'm calling fat.

I tried jogging recently and parts of my body screamed at me to stop, because it hurt. Then I realized my ankles and knees weren't the only body parts complaining. Where did my side start cramping? Up at my armpit? NO! Way down inside the roll of Badonk-adonk I have wrapped around my middle. Exactly what I want to get rid of. All my medications cause weight gain and the high calorific value of all gluten free products, mean depressive binge eating makes my jeans shrink.

I don't know how to get rid of these devils inhabiting many of us. I do know I need to start doing something to lose the weight. At my heaviest I have been 249 pounds. At my lightest I only weighed 7 pounds. When I married, I weighed 120. So by 2017 I was twice the man Ann married.

Oh look. There's a bar of Dairy Milk Chocolate — British Chocolate — no! Back! Leave me alone! Help! What do I do? I can't resist!

Oh, well. I thought about it.

If it is to be, it is up to me.

Even with the most positive of attitudes, I still have RSD and that will never change. Researchers are looking for a cure and ways to make the lives of sufferers easier. Right now, I must accept reality and make the most of it. I've found both with the pain I suffer and the pain our foster children have had to deal with, that generally, no one else can do it for me. No one else wants to and no one else cares enough. There is a cool statement I've seen in several books I've read, "**if it is to be, it is up to me.**" I've complained many times and in many situations that, if I don't do it, it doesn't happen.

Whether that's true or not, the idea of taking responsibility and acknowledging life is the way it is, is a good one.

Most of the bad things I've done, I did unwillingly, but *I* did them.

- *I* **was driving the car when we had the accident that killed Elizabeth and gave me RSD.**
- *I* **was cleaning the snow off the driveway, when I slipped and broke my ankle bones.**
- *I* **was getting the mail, when I slipped and cracked my skull.**
- *I* **was draining the camper's dirty water when I slipped and snapped the wrist bones off my right arm.**

And on and on through all the horrors I've gone through. The one constant is that I was present during all the traumas. Others were there for some of them. Some for many of them. The only one there for all of them was me. I remember that much about every one of them, I was definitely there. This means that I surely must have learned something from each of them happening, doesn't it?

The questions that need answering are:

- **Have *I* learned anything?**

- Am *I* able to accept what has happened, and get on with my life?
- Am *I* willing to accept responsibility for the way life is?

I should be able to answer yes to all the questions and, more importantly, be able and willing to update my plan of happiness so my spirit knows what to do when the questions need to be answered again. As well as accepting life is what it is and taking responsibility for my part in making it the way it is, there is also the idea that the roles I play have responsibilities that only I can fulfill.

An example of "if it is to be, it is up to me." and taking responsibility happened one January day for me.

06:49 Got up, got dressed; help children get ready.
07:45 Say prayers
07:50 Drive older children 8.6 miles south to school.
08:10 Head home, 8.6 miles north
08:25 Pick up littlest one to get her to preschool.
08:40 Arrive school, 8.4 miles north.
08:50 Leave school go to Ann's work to drop her off
as her car is off the road, 13.7 miles northwest
09:25 Drop Ann off and go home, 7.5 miles northeast
10:30 Leave home, having cleaned kitchen, washed dishes
and tidied. Head to school to take two children to the
dentist, 8.4 miles south
11:00 Leave school during a fire drill and head to dentist,
6.6 miles east.
11:30 Leave dentist, fetch the littlest one from pre- school.
11:37 Go home to get meat out for dinner and pick up
something a child forgot. 7.4 miles northwest
11:40 Leave home and head to pre-school. 6.6 miles north
11:52 Arrive at pre-school and collect daughter
11:58 Leave school, head back to the dentist, 13.7 miles
southeast
12:18 Arrive at dentist, make appointments

12:26 Take children back to school via, McDonald's, 6.6 miles west
01:05 Pick up a different child. Leave school and head home, 8.4 miles north
01:15 Arrive home
01:22 Leave for ACYI
01:49 Arrive ACYI via Seagull Book, 10.3 miles north
02:09 Head to Plain City to pick Ann up, 17.4 miles southeast
02:30 Arrive at Ann's school
02:48 Head to school to pick children up 4.6 miles west.
Major personal catastrophe occurs.
03:25 Arrive home, 8.4 miles north
04:10 Leave home to get child
04:25 Arrive ACYI, 9.8 miles. Pick up child.
04:37 Arrive home, 9.8 miles
05:00 Friends come to dinner and the day calms down.

In total, I drove 165 miles back and forth down the same road and all for other members of my family. At no point was I more than nine miles from home. Personally, I had a horrible day, full of pain and a catastrophe, yet I did what I did because someone needed to. The fact I felt like I had the flu, didn't stop me. I took responsibility.

When we're suffering with mental or physical anguish, there seems to be no joy or fun in what we're doing. When we realize everything was for our spouse and children, we begin to feel joyful, because we'd spent our time doing something useful. This wasn't only responsibility; this was service to my family and it gave me joy. A hole needed filling and I filled it. I didn't think about getting anything in return. As my family is the most important part of my life, I did what was important to me.

As I thought about what I was doing, my spirit bubble positively charged. I was giving service and my spirit bubble automatically filled with joy. The catastrophe was still trying to fill my bubble with pain and misery. I believe the joy won by a very small amount, but it won. The choice was simple; have a pity party, no one would come to, or get on with life and find joy.

Being complimentary

Who doesn't like being commended and complimented? This is one of the best ways to fill our spirit bubbles with positive emotions. Even when the other person has not been so nice to us, we can still find something to compliment them about. We may need to take a deep breath, or even several, and then return a minute or two later to give the compliment. Children thrive when we compliment them on their use of their talents. Their spirit bubbles fill to overflowing when they hear their parent's compliments. Unfortunately, they may say the opposite and it takes a lot of patience, as the parent, not to become upset. We have to then ensure we continue being complimentary even when others aren't doing the same.

A child practicing a musical instrument needs support, not having their parents complain about the awful din they are making. Children tend to believe what they are told. If they are being told they're no good, they will believe that they are no good

If they are told they are clever they will believe that they are clever, especially when they hear this a lot.

Negative things do not need to be said very often for them to believed. Many therapists argue that for each negative thing said, 5 positive things need saying to counterbalance.

I take every opportunity to tell my children how well they're doing as well as when they have room to improve. Pretending they are tremendous when they are average or even poor, actually does harm.

I try my hardest to compliment my children several times each day. I make sure I'm being honest and loving when doing so and I can testify my children blossom and grow. We all love compliments, but children need them so they can learn how to give them when they grow older and become parents.

Our spouse will also enjoy compliments from us. In many cases even ones that sound contrived can work. Like I love the way you made the bed this morning, said in the right tone of voice can have the desired effect. It also can deflect bad feelings.

My wife and children do tell me they don't like or need compliments. Their faces and body language make me disagree with them. I find that giving compliments makes me feel better. Doing so fills **my** spirit with positivity and this is how I am able to ignore the pain. Even if this wasn't so, I would still give compliments. If I wasn't suffering in the way I am with the constant chronic pain, I am confident that there would be other trials to deal with, where a positive spirit bubble would be essential.

If not parenthood, what is <u>your</u> most important role?

Some of you may disagree on the significance of being a parent and that is acceptable. After all, this is my opinion and you may have noticed I've gone out of my way to show this is what *I* believe.

If you disagree with me, I would be interested in knowing what is the most important role you feel you play in your life. Of course, some of us aren't parents and that's also okay. Let me know what you consider your most important role to be. Unless you're married you can't be a spouse and if you have no children you can't be a parent. If like me, you had an unmarried childless aunt and a childless aunt and uncle you can never be a cousin.

If, however, we're married and have children then spouse and parent are roles you play whether we value the role or not. There are too many single parent families where the parent is **not** a widow or widower. This unfortunately shows the role of parent isn't as important to these people as **I** believe it should be. I can't comprehend this attitude or work out what they consider more important.

If we have no family members, if we are an orphan then family is a concept that we will have difficulty with. I know of a person who was adopted as an orphan and when her parents divorced neither wanted to take her with them. She asked if we could adopt her, so she could have a family to come home to during college holidays. Without a family she would not even have a home to go home to. We seriously considered adopting her as we couldn't stand the thought of her having nobody.

I don't know what happened to her because the accident intervened and she had aged out of the foster care system by the time we had recovered. We were unable to find out where she had gone and CPS weren't interested in helping us find her. I hope she found a wonderful man and started a family of her own. I know there is nothing I can do about it if she hasn't.

I have many other roles I play as well, it is just that, for me, husband is my #1 and fatherhood is my #2. Both of these roles allow me to show that most elusive emotion to define – love. The other familial roles also allow me to show love. The other roles, in my opinion, allow me to fulfill my responsibilities towards my family.

What is love?

What is love? This is a question asked thousands of times a day for thousands of years. Often by the same person trying to work out whether their boyfriend or girlfriend really is someone they can love and will love them. An Internet search returns millions of hits on the topic. Most provide the following list.

- Eros or Erotic Love.
- Agape or Selfless Love.
- Philia or Affectionate Love
- Storge or familiar Love
- Ludus or Playful Love.
- Mania or Obsessive Love
- Pragma or Enduring Love.
- Philautia or Self Love

I have to admit that I didn't realize there were so many variations of love for us to consider. I also admit that I have never heard of most of them.

I'm going with the Apostle Paul from the New Testament and his definition of love as found in 1 Corinthians 13. Love suffers long and doesn't look forward to the child's 18th birthday so they can be kicked out of the family home. I'm not sure how many children who have had this happen have actually been upset at being kicked out. They will obviously be upset that they have nowhere to live. Love bears all things, believes all things, hopes all things, and endures all things. Love never fails. This list should show our love for our spouse and our children is overarching. It should be the primary, central purpose of our lives and the key to having any success.

The rock in the back of the picture is the Rock of Gibraltar. It has been there for millennia and will stay there for as long. It is part of the Pillars of Hercules at the entrance to the Mediterranean Sea. It is something fixed and immovable as, I believe, should be our love for others, especially when the "others" are our family members. The Rock could become unfixed and movable, but it would take some big bombs and an awful lot of effort channeled in the wrong direction. The

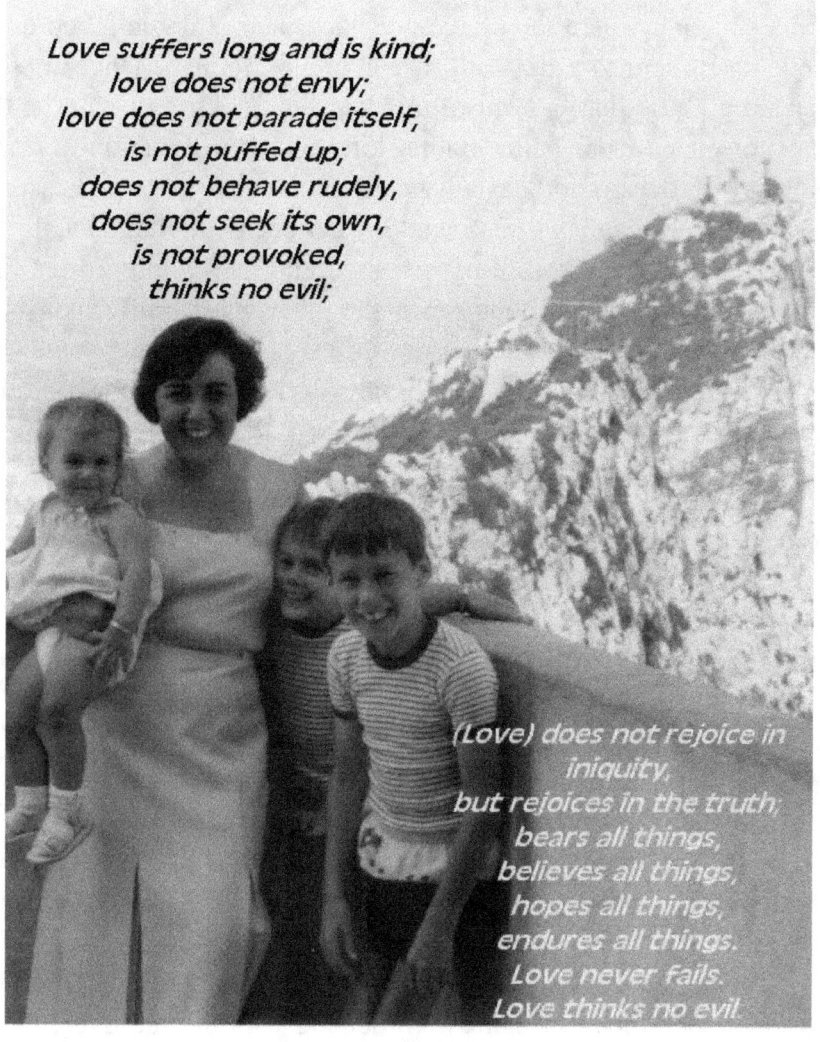

Love suffers long and is kind;
love does not envy;
love does not parade itself,
is not puffed up;
does not behave rudely,
does not seek its own,
is not provoked,
thinks no evil;

(Love) does not rejoice in
iniquity,
but rejoices in the truth;
bears all things,
believes all things,
hopes all things,
endures all things.
Love never fails.
Love thinks no evil.

179

same is true for our family relationships. It takes a lot of energy channeled in the wrong direction to destroy.

Don't judge

I believe this is how we should deal with everyone. For example, Ann has taught me that the mothers of our foster children, as daughters of God, deserve to be treated as He would. This seems to me to be a good way of looking at things. We generally have no idea what has led to the situation where they have poisoned their children's bodies and condemned them to a life full of pain and suffering. Many times, it's their drug abuse that has led to this happening. The question is, does that prevent us from being polite, kind and generous anyway? Ann thinks that it doesn't and has always taken the time to be as pleasant as she could when dealing with them. She has been non-judgmental.

I'm a normal person, a normal man and my children often drive me bonkers, up the wall and down the other side. I suffer constantly with pain that can be made worse with the stress of being somewhere between the top and bottom of the wall. This doesn't mean I can judge others, even the biological parents of my children.

Assume the best

To help myself, I assume the best possible version of what my child just said or did and believe no evil has occurred. This means always doing my best to avoid shouting at them or speaking using an unpleasant voice. With teenagers, this is difficult as it can be almost impossible not to respond in kind. It is a "nail jelly to a tree" or "herding cats" sort of situation.

Many of us seem to do the opposite of "thinks no evil" and come into a situation having prejudged it and to some extent have been judge, jury and executioner, even before we know the facts. We make negative assumptions, not just about our children but about others in society.

Think about how that sounds to our children. There can be many reasons we do this, especially wen dealing with our teenage children. With a teenager, a simple question such as, 'How was your day?" can

180

be responded to in a tone that should only be used when speaking to someone who has just tried to kill you. Asking them to do some sort of chore like hanging up the towel they just used and we are spoken to in an even more unpleasant tone of voice that includes shouting.

My method is to respond in a calm quiet voice. I still often get shouted at and verbally abused in response to the simplest of statements or questions, delivered in the most loving tone I can manage. I admit that I often fail to use my most loving voice, but I intend to keep on trying.

Is it easy? Not at all, in fact it is one of the hardest things to do. Nuclear physics and flying the Space shuttle are actually much easier tasks than dealing with teenage children. The knowledge that they will either grow out of it or get married makes it no easier to handle. Still, we have to do our best. One of my children sent me a text telling me that now she had reached 25 years old and was a mother herself that she realized I was "right all the time."

Our family aren't the only ones who may think evil of us. Our friends and associates can also do so. This often happens when, for some inexplicable reason, they think we do nothing good, nothing right and think evil of them constantly. They use this as justification for why they respond to everything we say and do in a negatively.

We can be like them in our responses or we can show we're adults, intent on showing love knows no evil. We'll keep our spirit bubbles full of joy and happiness and allow our positivity to suck the negativity out of their bubbles. We'll fight the pain they may be causing us, or the pain we suffer that has nothing to do with them and find joy.

Get on with it all.

Get on with it! Sounds easy because it's only three words, It isn't, it's one of the hardest truths to deal with. Sometimes, life gets better. At other times, it doesn't. With me, things didn't and haven't. My life has continued at its headlong downward pace and catastrophes, of one sort or another, continue to occur at the rate of 1 to 3 per month. It snows and the central heating breaks. The air conditioning had broken during the hottest days of summer. It broke when a power surge blew out the capacitor. The same surge set the mountain on fire and burned a hundred acres behind our house. Replacing a $20 capacitor seems insignificant in comparison.

Catching a break, apart from an impossible expression, doesn't seem possible for any of us. The term means to get some relief, or to make something less severe for a time. Others want to catch a break themselves and we're all running around with our butterfly nets, hoping to catch an elusive creature called a break. This is as easy to do as catching a snipe.

I find prayer helps me immensely even if, for some reason, my prayers to have a burden lifted have only made me more capable of handling the burden. I pray daily I can make it through the day, even with RSD, and can do what I need to do. You know what? It works! I posted this to Facebook in 2015.

Ok, it's 1015 and so far today I have helped get the children to school, blown the tire up on Ann's car, hung Olivia's clothes up, put a new pump on the furnace so we now have central heating again, cleaned up the mess from the septic system backing up again, prayed I'd flushed whatever was blocking it, fixed the step on the patio the dog managed to knock off, helped Amy with a programming question on Excel. Washed a load of dishes and put them away. Fixed two kitchen cupboards, which will hopefully stay fixed now. Oh, and I fixed the handle on the door to the garage so it doesn't come off in your hand anymore. And, I'm in as much pain now as I was at 7am when I got up.

Could I have managed without prayer? Possibly. I know I succeeded because of it. I was unable to do much for the next few days, because I hurt. However, this day I was successful and for this, I'm grateful. This cycle is how I live my life. I overdo it and hurt a lot the next day. I take time to recover, which may be a few days or even only one. I then overdo it again. For me, pain free doesn't mean I am in no pain. These sorts of days don't occur. A pain free day is one where the level of pain I'm in, is lower than level I can manage. Prayer helps me to smile and be happy, although I do warn people to be careful of this sort of blessing.

Self-defeating

When life gets worse, it can be because we expect it to. A fit, healthy person, whose life is the way they want it to be, can easily find something to complain about. I know I did before RSD turned my life upside down. A good six-figure salary with perks and benefits and heading for a 7-figure salary and yet, I could complain. This tells me an excellent job, money, being fit and healthy and not having too many problems, didn't stop me from being self-defeating. I now have no job, am far from fit, and often find I have less to complain about.

Whatever the situation we find ourselves in; we have excuses or reasons for not acting. We can complain we don't get chances or any number of reasons we can't. Remember excuses and reasons aren't the same. An excuse is used to avoid doing something we **don't want to do**. A reason is why **we can't do it**.

When I taught at a college, I'd hear some good excuses. "I did badly on the final because I fell asleep last night while revising." 100% attendance was needed for several classes to get an A. The excuses weren't original or even interesting and were generally to do with self-defeating behavior.

If it is to be, it is up to me, needs us to accept reasons, but that we kick excuses to the touchline. I've found it is up to me, because I'm the only one who controls the way I feel and I'm the only one I have any control over when it comes to emotions. I can upset others very quickly and easily, but they control how they deal with it.

I don't want to upset anyone, but as you doubtless know, it is hard to avoid doing so. One thing I can do is to accept that if it is to be it is up to me and take the high road. For example, we can apologize even when we feel we aren't in the wrong. We can do it when it is very difficult to do – when everyone knows we aren't in the wrong. We can

183

make sure we apologize first. I've learned from parenting 130+ children how easy it is to upset them. I always take the opportunity to compliment my children; I thank them for what they have done when they have completed their chores and I have learned to quickly apologize when I have upset them.

I apologize for a number of reasons; the most important one being to teach them we are never too high and mighty to say "I'm sorry" when we have made a mistake even if it is to someone who is only 5-years-old at the time.

Don't negatively charge our children's spirit bubbles

Not apologizing teaches our children that the "law of the west" is ***"do as I say, not as I do."*** We are teaching them that the weaker person in a relationship has no choice but to apologize and the stronger person in the relationship does not.

I could argue that I am in constant, chronic, mind bending pain and therefore get a pass. Or I give them everything they have and that makes it acceptable for me to ignore the Golden Rule. I could come up with dozens of reasons, but they are really just excuses.

What we are really saying is that it is our right, our heritage to be able to forcibly fill your spirit bubble with as much negativity as we can. There is nothing you can do about it, kid, so just suck it up. You will get to do it when you get your own children, but right now I am in charge, OK.?

Is that true, is that what we really are all about? Or more likely we have just allowed ourselves into being like that over time; maybe because we're lazy or possibly because we're stressed.

When we realize this is what is happening, don't dwell on the problem. Don't psycho-analyze yourself and try to work out why you are doing it. Simply put a stake in the ground and say, "No more. From today, I am going to positively charge my children's spirit bubbles." We must tell ourselves we are going to do this regardless of the disbelief we will receive from our children; regardless of the fact they will continue to act badly until they do believe us.

Parenting is a full time job that can fill our spirit bubbles with joy as long as we work at making it so.

Mr. Mum

If pain and sorrow and total punishment immediately followed the doing of evil, no soul would repeat a misdeed. If joy and peace and rewards were instantaneously given the doer of good, there could be no evil–all would do good and not because of the rightness of doing good. There would be no test of strength, no development of character, no growth ....
(Spencer W. Kimball)

As Spencer Kimball says in the above quote we are basically a work in progress, learning as we go how strong we are and what a wonderful person we are. We learn how to keep our spirit bubbles filled with positivity as we do so. We will get it wrong, and putting it right, is how we learn and grow. We may have to study hard to see how some events make us grow; but I can safely guarantee that they did. Personally, I try to look back on my experiences and find someway of turning it into a pleasant or humorous memory.

One experience I had makes me laugh every time I think about it. I don't need to run the "tickle my amygdala" app, to get the same response.

The year is 1987 and I'm doing my impression of Arthur Dent, from Douglas Adams novel, Hitchhikers Guide to the Galaxy. I'd not shaved for three or four days, so I had a scruffy beard. I'd been in hospital for those three days and had not bathed either, so my hair was a mess. I had on a pair of cotton pajamas, a dressing gown and a pair of slippers. I was also alone in the OBGYN suite of my local hospital sitting in a wheelchair, waiting in line, with a bunch of pregnant women, outside of an ultrasound suite.

So, you understand how and why I'm there, I need to give you some background information. I hope you're sufficiently intrigued at why I was posing as a pregnant man, to stay with me.

186

My two eldest children, Simon and Andrew are handicapped and when they were little, we'd go to a specially fitted out school classroom on a Saturday morning, once a month. Everything, except the ceiling, was covered in soft play foam cushion material. It was a safe place for handicapped children, because when they fell, the ground was soft. There was a floor to ceiling slide, made from the soft play material and dozens of pieces left lying around, perfect for throwing at each other. In the middle, there was a padded balance beam.

It was also a fun place for a 30+ dad to play in. I was the only parent who spent time in the playroom. All the other parents spent their time in another classroom, where there was tea, coffee and cookies, I spent no time in the chat room and no other parent ever joined me in the playroom. Each time, I'd spend all morning running around and throwing pieces of foam at the children. I'd also gently throw some of the children around onto the soft play equipment. I didn't know it at the time, but I was filling my spirit bubble with joy, while also positively charging the children's bubbles. My children have the memories and they can replay them.

All the children, not only mine, loved to be pushed over and thrown into the piles of foam. I enjoyed it and got a lot of exercise. I also enjoyed myself immensely. I realized early on in my career as a father, I could do most of what my children can, even when I'm classified as too old. The soft play area wasn't the only place I've been able to play with my children, on equipment limited to the younger generation. Its a great reason to be a father.

Record number of children

As I write this, Ann and I have had 130+ children and I still get the opportunity to play with my little ones in places meant for people 50 or more years younger than I am. We will return to 1987 and my visit to the OBGYN suite shortly and then find out whether I was pregnant. How quickly depends on how fast a reader you are.

Right now, we're heading to the Internet, to do some research and find the record for the most children. The Guinness Book of Records shows the world record for the most children officially recorded is 69, by the first of two wives of Feodor Vassilyev (1707-1782).

He was a peasant from Shuya, 150 miles east of Moscow. In 27 confinements, Mrs. Vassilyev gave birth to 16 pairs of twins, 7 sets of triplets and 4 sets of quadruplets. The children were born between 1725 and 1765.

For some reason, the poor woman's first name isn't in the record books. Merely that she was Feodor Vassilyev's first wife. I can't believe she even let her husband into the same house as her, after the first few pregnancies. He had a further 18 children, 6 sets of twins and 2 sets of triplets with his 2nd wife. A total of 87 children. In 1782, when he died, 82 of his children were still alive.

96 children!

A man not in the Guinness Book of Records called Daad Mohammed Murad Abdul Rahman apparently has had 96 children. To reach this number, the retired truck driver has had 17 wives, most of whom he has divorced, as Islam has a limit of four wives at a time.

In 2012, he was preparing to divorce at least one of his current three wives, so he could marry two new ones, in his bid to reach his target of 100 children by 2015, at which time he would be 68 years old.

The last report I can find is dated May 2016 and says his eldest child is 49 years old and the youngest 16 months old. Even though he has divorced 17 wives, most still live with him. He was at 96 children and 74 grandchildren and hopes to reach 100 children by 2018.

Somewhere along the way, he has lost a leg. The news reports in the Arab Emirates newspaper don't say whether this has had any effect upon his childbearing abilities. Apparently not! I personally think he's cheating and Mrs. Vassilyev's one woman re-population record can't be broken.

Why Ann isn't in the record books

Ann isn't in the Guinness Book of Records instead of Mrs. Vassilyev, even though she's had more children, because there are many differences between the arrival of our 1st baby and our 100th baby. The major one is that Ann carried our 1st, Simon in her womb and our 100th, Dee, arrived by car. Unlike poor Mrs. Vassilyev, for most of our children, Ann has had no pregnancy issues to deal with, no labor pains, no cravings, and no weight gain.

Our 100th baby was a month old when she was delivered to our home, by a social worker from CPS. He pulled on to our drive, got out of his car and opened the rear passenger door. He took a baby seat out and put it onto the driveway, got back into his car saying, "I think it's a girl" and left. This method of delivery was unique; normally they at least came into the house, but he was on emergency call and needed to get back to the office.

This means I've only had to deal with all the vicissitudes of being the husband of a pregnant wife 5 of the 130+ times. The women among you will be, shaking your head at me. You men will know what I mean. This is another reason I can't understand how Feodor managed it, as his wife must have been, at the least, cranky when she realized she was pregnant yet again.

Our children have come to live with us, ranging in age from newborn to fifteen years old. Some have stayed with us for a fleeting time and some have stayed permanently, as we've adopted six. The largest number of children living with us at any time, since we started fostering in 1991, has been eleven and the lowest number has been three. If you find children annoying, our house isn't the place for you. We have five children in our home now, and noisy is an apt adjective for us. On school mornings, barely organized chaos is what you will often get. On others, you quickly realize 'quiet' is a relative term.

Back to 1987

When we left the story of my 1987 pregnancy, Ann and I had three children, two of whom are handicapped. I was in a soft-play room, where all handicapped children were welcome, including

189

mentally handicapped and children with Downs Syndrome. A child, who we will call Julian, caused me to finish off waiting my turn for an ultra sound, with some pregnant women.

One of the best activities was throwing the foam cubes, triangles, circles etc. at each other. They varied in size from 12-inch cubes to pieces 3 to 4 feet wide. Even the larger pieces didn't hurt when they hit us. They might knock us off our feet, but the ground was soft and so that was ok.

Julian was six feet in both directions and built solidly, so the cubes or triangles he threw hurt. If you get a hug from a Downs child, breathe in and stick your chest and stomach out as far as you can, so when the bear hug comes, you can breathe out and can keep breathing until they release you. They're hard to convince to do anything, so it takes some time.

When I had Downs Syndrome children in the playroom with me, I was extra careful. There were a few simple rules to follow, the most important of which was knowing where they were and what they were doing. I'd also talk to them a lot, to convince them to be gentle with the other children. This day I didn't keep an eye on where Julian was. As it turned out, he was behind me.

Can I fly?

Julian loved to throw the cubes around, except this day he decided to throw something a lot heavier, me. He picked me up and threw me ten feet across the room and against the balance beam. He threw me with enough force, I hit the metal bar under the padding hard. I made a thudding sound as I bounced and fell over. I couldn't get up for 10 minutes and lay there groaning.

As a consultant, I used the thud factor with reports I wrote for my clients. They had to have a thud factor, when dropped on the desk of the person for whom I was working. The louder the thud, the better the report was. I was thudded enough to finish off in the emergency room,

They admitted me to the hospital and put me in a room with a "nil by mouth" sign above the bed, in case they needed to do surgery. A doctor started attaching a drip into the back of my hand. Up until this time, I hated needles. They scared me for a common reason. I remembered vaccinations as a child and the memories were all painful. My plan of happiness told my spirit to avoid needles at all costs.

Nitty Nora

Those of you who were born in the mid to late 1950s may remember the joy of vaccinations. For us, a doctor came and each class of victims was lined up outside a room. The first time, the first person had no idea what was about to happen. The next child, and all later children, knew exactly what was coming. The child at the head of the line would go into the room, the door closed behind them, and eventually we were next. In my school, Nitty Nora, the dickey explorer, would grab us in her iron grip and pull our sleeve up. Using her sadistic voice, which she thought was kind, friendly and loving, she'd lie to us. "Relax, this won't hurt!" she'd say. Of course, she meant she'd feel no pain. If we were stressed and the needle wouldn't go in, she'd insist we relax. Her voice became even more friendly and scary.

Occasionally, we got the polio vaccine in a sugar cube. The relief was palpable; there was no screaming. The next time, however, we'd have our hopes dashed and Nitty Nora would have her steel gauntlets on. Sometimes, Nitty Nora would only want to check our head for lice. We were then set up for the next attack of the invading needles. If we did have head lice, we had the thrill of going home with a note telling our parents we had nits and instructions on how to deal with them.

A drip with a drip

These wonderful childhood memories have stayed with me and here I was, having a drip put in. At least that was the plan. My doctor must have slept through his phlebotomy class, or had someone else take the final test. His name badge should have read Doctor Ineptitude or Doctor Drip. He took several attempts to find a vein, poking me all over my hand, without once finding anything remotely like a blood vessel. The nurse watched him mess up, then pushed him to one side, inserted the needle into a vein, and connected the drip.

No one came back to check and a while later; the saline bag was half-full of my blood. I called for a nurse and she attached a new bag of saline solution. As weird as this sounds, this experience made me no longer fear needles and I even donate blood on a regular basis.

The doctors couldn't work out what had happened; what hurt so badly and so we embarked on a series of tests. Eventually, they decided Julian had thrown me with enough force to damage my liver, but they needed to do an ultra sound to be sure. As the only ultra sound machine available was at the maternity suite, they put me in a wheelchair and off we went. They omitted to tell me where we were headed, so I was unprepared. In fact, during my stay at the hospital they forgot to tell me what was happening most of the time.

Arthur Dent?

I'd been in the hospital for three or four days and, as I told you earlier, I hadn't shaved and had a scruffy beard. I hadn't bathed either, so my hair was a mess. I was wearing a pair of cotton pajamas, a dressing gown and a pair of slippers. If you know Douglas Adams *Hitchhikers Guide to the Galaxy*, you'll realize I looked like Arthur Dent. The only thing I was missing was my towel.

This was the last of a series of tests I underwent. The day before, I'd had x-rays, using barium. They gave me a jug with 160 fluid ounces of aniseed-flavored water and a two-ounce cup. They told me to drink a cupful every 10 minutes. After a couple of hours and many little cups, my bladder was complaining. I asked a nurse if they needed a full bladder for the test.

While I waited for her to find out, the sun went nova, a new one had gone through half of its life cycle, and I'd drunk several more cupfuls of evil fluid. She returned to say no, my bladder didn't need to be full. I waddled gratefully to the nearest bathroom and sat down on the toilet. I can't show you how a grateful waddle looks in print. I'm sure you can imagine how I looked. As the pressure was so great, nothing improved. I took several minutes to start peeing. Once I did, the sun had the chance to go through a lot more life cycle. If I'd been with some boy scouts, I could have put a bonfire out by myself.

Sonogram, please

Today, they'd given me no more details of what they'd planned for me. No one had told me where they were taking me, only to put on my dressing gown and slippers. My morphine drip and I got in an ambulance and had a ride across the hospital. I initially had no idea I was on the maternity suite. As I looked around, I saw all the other waiting patients were pregnant women. They were all giving me confused looks, whispering to each other, and nodding or pointing towards me. The nurses called someone's name such as "Mrs. Smith" and a woman, in some stage of pregnancy, would go into the room. After several women had been called, I realized where I was and why. I had not developed the tool of chatting to anyone and everyone, so I sat there silently. CT and MRI technology wasn't available yet so this was the only choice available.

Then the nurse came out and made all the pregnant women's jaws drop. "Mr. Gray." she called. I raised my hand and she came over to wheel me into the ultra sound suite. The women couldn't believe their eyes. There was no way I could be mistaken for an ugly woman. I stayed in the wheelchair, so they couldn't see my belly. Today, I have the big belly, but I didn't in 1985. I developed it after this experience. I didn't get to wait around afterwards, but it would have been fun to find out what they thought was happening.

The ultra sound was inconclusive and so the doctor told me he wanted to do a liver function test. I'd no idea what he meant, so he showed me what looked like a large knitting needle with a grabbing tool on the end and a plunger at the top. He told me that, using a local anesthetic, he'd poke the needle into my side, push the plunger and snip a piece of liver off to test.

The size of the needle was such I blanched and the next day, the pain stopped and my side turned black, blue, yellow and green. Up until then, there had been no bruising, no evidence I'd been hurt, except for the increased doses of morphine I'd been taking. The doctors decided my flying lesson had damaged my liver and, as I no longer hurt, I could go home

Reliving the past with joy

You may wonder how telling this story isn't returning to the point on the mountain where the trauma occurred. As I enjoy telling the experience and I don't get upset when I do, I believe there's no problem. I'm retelling what happened at that point in my journey. I can only do this, if I can look at the event dispassionately and I can.

If I want to use the experience as an example of how life is unkind to me, I'm heading down the 'victim mentality' side road. I get joy and pleasure looking back at the many elements of humor from the experience. At the time, I hurt. Now, though, I can replay what happened in my mind and laugh. I also recall I damaged my liver and when I recently had blood tests and my liver numbers were elevated 1000%, I initially blamed this accident. When the numbers kept increasing, we could discard that possibility. When they came down into the normal range because we knew I had Celiac's disease and was eating gluten free food, it was obvious my rag doll experience had no lasting effect.

I've no control over the fact the pain I'm suffering is staying, but my ability to find joy in what happened and laugh about it, **that** I choose and I fill my spirit bubble with positive energy.

Dispassion or dat passion?

If you've experienced trauma, psychologists will want you to revisit the memory with the aim of learning to look dispassionately, unemotionally and objectively. Realize that, even if it was all our fault, what happened some miles back up the road, no longer has any control over our life.

- *Accept we can't go back and make it un-happen.*

194

- *We can refuse to allow it to keep us idling on the edge of the road.*
- *We can write the experience down in our journal. We could also write it on a piece of paper then burn it.*
- *We can turn it into a humorous anecdote as I do.*
- *We can write a letter to the person who offended us, or who hurt us, tell them what we think of them, and tell them we have decided to get on with our life anyway. We're not going to allow them to keep us from moving on; they aren't worth it. Many experts will tell us <u>NOT</u> to send the letter. We're to destroy it and let the bad feelings go as well.*

You can probably come up with several ideas yourself. You'll also realize all these ideas take real effort on our part. Problems, difficulties, tribulations, whatever we want to call them have a positive side to them. Each makes us grow. Writing a letter to the person who hurt us takes time and nerve if we're going to send it.

A friend talked with a therapist about some trauma that had occurred nearly 30 years earlier and they stupidly recommended the letter be sent. The can of worms this opened for both the victim and the abuser caused a lot of anger and some resentment. I personally recommended the letter be burned.

Whatever we do to let go of the hurt it will take a lot of effort. We need to do it, because otherwise we are stuck in the victim mentality side road. If we spend too much time there, there is every possibility that it will be immensely difficult to get out. If you have ever had a snowplow throw the snow from the road onto your driveway, you'll know how difficult it can become to get out.

Another friend says he doesn't have trials, he sees them as life happening. His philosophy is to resolve a problem and wait for the next one. I'm not sure I agree with him, especially if multiple learning experiences all come at the same time, but he is happy because it works for him.

Act or be acted upon

One thing my friend is correct about is the concept of **act or be acted upon**. The RSD acts upon me. I get to choose how I act about having RSD. I am acted upon by the pain and other than remembering to take my medications, there is nothing I can do. If I forget to take them it's disastrous and by noon I can do nothing.

I take my medications and can **act as if** I am in a lot less pain than I really am. Granted, when I over do it, I have to pay for this decision and take it easy for the next few days. Even then, I have the satisfaction of knowing something that needed doing got done.

Whether we wish to act or be acted upon is a personal choice. My son was unlucky enough to get pleurisy in June 2017. This painful condition can only be resolved with bed rest, pain killers and steroids. Unfortunately, the pain killers are strong enough to fit the category of "no pain, no brain". The pain is gone, but so is our brain and we can get lots of bed rest. In this situation, my son spent several days being acted upon. Everything he needed, someone else had to provide.

When we are acted upon we are allowing others to do what we should be doing. When we act, we are obviously providing for ourselves. I have this choice. I can take medicines to a level the pain has gone but so has my brain. I could then leave the problem of dealing with my physical body to others. I would then be acted upon in everything. I choose to act by taking enough pain medications that I am able to keep thinking.

There are many areas of our lives where we have no choice over being acted upon. Most of our dealings with the governments of the town, county, state, country we live in, leave us acted upon. Even then we have the ability to act. We are being acted upon when the governments set the speed limits on roads, we get to choose and act by observing these limits. If we chose to disregard them we will be acted upon by a police officer giving us a speeding ticket. This will cause us emotional and spiritual pain as well as whatever type of pain the loss of money is.

Acting, either in the concept of acting as if the situation was as we would like it to be; or when there is nothing we can do about the situation, is often a test of our strength of will. At other times we can decide whether what we are doing doesn't seem to work. That could be a time to a time to try something different.

When we act and become agents for ourselves we will find that agents have more power than those who wait to be acted upon. Those people cannot choose to become better and can't progress down the road. They are stuck in one of the side canyons on their journey down the mountain. They get acted upon and are at the mercy of everything else. They have dark, negative spirit bubbles.

I choose to act; to be agent for my own pain management; I choose to ignore the pain as best I can; I choose to become better and always have a positively charged spirit bubble.

I choose **not** to be a rock on the mountain road, acted upon by the wind and the rain, never achieving anything useful. My objective is to have a spirit bubble full of joy and to fight pain and find joy. All of my goals and choices short-term or long-term should be helping me to achieve that objective. A rock on the side of the mountain is not my objective.

Who nose when we'll move

Happiness isn't in the mere possession of money; it lies in the joy of achievement, in the thrill of creative effort.
(Franklin D. Roosevelt)

Talking of being acted upon, reminds me of a time I didn't think through what I was doing. I have no idea whether the British Railway companies still use the train carriages I used to travel home from the bank I worked at in the City of London in the 1970s. Each carriage was divided into separate sub carriages, which had two six-seater bench seats and a door on each side. Once you had chosen the sub carriage, you stayed there until the next station.

I lived 35 miles from the City of London and 20 miles from the final station. The train began full but, I was often alone by the time we reached my station and I'd fall asleep. I generally managed to wake before my station. If I didn't, I'd get off at the next one and catch a train headed the opposite way. This day I was woken when the train coming to a sudden, shuddering stop.

Alone and bored

I pulled the door window down and looked along the train, to see if I could figure out why and where we stopped. I was near the back and could see, off in the distance, the engine. We were stationary, nearly a half mile outside of a station, but I couldn't tell which one. Every few minutes, I'd open a window and peer out. Without a station platform, it was too far to jump to the tracks, not that I wanted to. I may have been a relatively fit young man, but the idea of hiking to the station didn't appeal to me, and it was illegal.

198

I kept looking to relieve the boredom. Technology has come a long way in the last 40 years. In 1974, there were no cell phones, no personal computers, no laptops or anything even remotely similar. The bank I worked for ran their whole business on a computer with 196k of memory. It had several banks of 5mb hard disks, each the size of a washing machine. My current phone has 3.2 million times the disk space on a disk 0.5 square inches. I'd taken no books with me to read on the train that day, so I was stuck.

The last time I opened the window, turned out to have devastating consequences. The train jerked forward and I was thrown a few inches back. The window came slamming up, connecting with the bottom of my nose. I fell backwards onto a seat, where I lay, crying from the discomfort. There was no one to commiserate me; nor were there any other males there to mock or deride me. I was 18, and although this wasn't my first broken bone, up to that time it was the most painful.

All alone, bored and no girls

I don't believe, even had there been many beautiful girls present, I'd have been unable to avoid crying. I'd previously broken my nose when playing soccer. The goalkeeper kicked the ball straight at my face. The ball bounced back over his head and into the goal. That was nowhere near as painful as the window, and at least I scored a goal.

The train pulled into what turned out to be the final station on the line. Holding on to my horribly battered and bruised nose, I staggered onto the other platform, and onto a train heading back toward London. I want you to find joy in any pain you're suffering, but please stop laughing at my calamity. When I eventually got home, it didn't hurt as much. I doubt I'd have gotten any sympathy anyway, as my parents were both in the medical profession and it had to be hanging off to get any sympathy from them.

As normal, there was no joy in the experience.

I didn't have a girl looking after me. The joy comes from retelling the story. Most people laugh when I tell them what happened and I join in the laughter. I learned to lean on the train window in the future. I wasn't a victim of anything other than bad luck and being somewhere there was a gremlin looking for mischief. There is generally nothing we can do if the gremlins are determined to get us. This doesn't really happen that often as they prefer to work alone.

Catastrophes

Poor decisions can have catastrophic results and we may pay for them a lot longer than I suffered with my broken nose, which hurt for two weeks. I still have problems, even though it is no longer broken. Generally, these problems aren't as painful as having a broken nose.

My foster son, Darius, and his biological, physician father are an example of someone doing something he may have done before, with no consequences. He did it one more time and, this time, the consequences were heartbreaking. Dad figuratively drove off the mountain road completely, when he made a terrible choice and shook his two-month-old son for crying. I know he had a momentary lapse of judgment. He didn't intend to shake Darius so violently; he gave him shaken baby syndrome. Darius was left with a huge lump on his skull and permanent, severe brain damage. Father was a doctor and knew the result, yet he did it. His choice cost him a lot, as the police rightly held him responsible for his stupid choice. He lost his freedom and his career. His wife lost her son, her husband, her sense of security and possibly all she had.

I have come to collect some breast milk

His mother was still feeding him and I had to make several visits to the CPS office to collect expressed milk to feed him with, until we weaned him over to formula. This made for some carefully phrased requests, when I arrived at the office. The receptionists, especially those who knew me, gave me some odd looks when I told them I was there to collect some breast milk. Naturally, I'd spent some time on the journey to the office trying to come up with new and embarrassing ways to phrase my request. This is another time I wish I'd had a video camera turned on. The looks on the women's faces was priceless, except for the ones who knew why I was there, who burst into laughter at the shocked facial expressions of the other women. I chose to make sure I asked someone I hadn't previously met to ensure my spirit bubble would be filled with joy from the experience.

Blankie therapy

We learned an important lesson with Darius, regarding how to help when life is too much. I was in the car, outside of a store, waiting for Ann to come out. Darius was in his car seat behind me. He'd dropped his blankie and was screaming, so I reached over and threw the blankie towards him. It fell over his head and he went quiet. I got out the car and removed the blankie and he started bawling again. Intrigued. I put the blanket back over his head and he stopped crying. With the blanket over his head, no stimuli were reaching his brain and this was calming him down. We have used this knowledge many times in the years since. It can be better to remove a child from the situation, than to leave them in it, when they're over stimulated. Taking them out for a few minutes to catch their breath, gives them the opportunity to regain control of themselves, even when they are babies.

Darius came to us because he needed lots of attention. Unfortunately, we were unable to do anything for him, beyond giving him tender loving care and covering his eyes, when everyday life became too much for him. He was one of our foster children we have no idea what happened to. He moved to a critical care medical home, so he could get the constant care he needed. Shaken baby syndrome is a spur of the moment, lose your temper issue with long-term consequences.

When teaching our children, we explain there are consequences to our actions. Some can be catastrophic as Darius and his parents found. His father was jailed for child abuse. His mother may have sacrificed a lot for medical school and now all was lost from one moment of anger. They both lost their son, who they must have loved. I can't see how they ever put their lives together again. I hope they did and that Darius somehow overcame his problems. I unfortunately have to admit I can see no way he possibly could have. That sort of truama is permanent and there is no cure.

No ticket

The consequence of my stupidity with the train window was only to hurt to myself. No one else got hurt. 20 years later, though, it saved me from a speeding ticket.

I broke my nose a third time, when I stepped in front of a moving bus and left a nose track down the windows. I was lucky I only broke my nose. In a 3-year period ending in 2015, 23 people were killed in the same area I snotted up the bus. The broken septum, the cartilage in the middle of the nose, was making it hard to breathe through my nose, giving me sleep apnea. I had surgery to straighten the septum, and the doctors had packed my nose with bandage and given me a metal nose guard to wear. They also gave me two black eyes. The cop took one look at me, changed his attitude, and told me to be more careful in the future.

On a side note, the amount of packing a doctor can get up a nose is truly amazing. When the doctor pulled the bandages out, it was like watching a magician. I remember wondering how much more there could possibility be and when would he stop, because it hurt. Unfortunately, once he had finished on one nostril, he repeated the exercise on the other one. It likely only took a couple of minutes, it felt like hours. I can't speak for you, but from personal experience, I must admit I appear to have an empty head.

More surgery

Both operations to fix my nose were done under general anesthetic. The first surgery had tried to straighten the septum, without fixing the external bones. This second was to try to do both. They straightened the septum, but simply moved the break bump a half inch down my nose.

To reset a bone it generally needs re-breaking it and that guaranteed I wouldn't have kept still. I know this from an earlier experience with surgery on my face. I was born with a large cyst over my right eye. For some reason, I was 16-years-old before the surgery to remove it was scheduled. The surgeon told me they needed to pop my eye, cut the cyst out, stitch the hole closed and pop the eyeball back in. I was glad to have a general anesthetic.

He also told me he'd had a similar operation, where they popped his eye out under a local anesthetic. He'd wanted to watch the procedure and they gave him a mirror. I didn't check if he was telling the truth, as the last thing I remember is reaching five or six on the count to ten and I never see him again.

When I came to, I was numb for the first 10 of so minutes and couldn't understand why I couldn't see. I couldn't feel the bandages and I was worried I'd gone blind. Not long after I worked out there was a bandage covering both eyes, a nurse came and removed it.

My father decided to remove the stitches a week or so later. He came at me, with what seemed to me to be pair of stitch cutters big enough to cut ornamental hedge animals. Naturally I backed off, but finished off backed into a corner, where he removed the stitches, which only took 2 seconds, or 5 minutes in elapsed time.

I was therefore happy to have the surgeries on my nose under general anesthetic. My eye surgery occurred in the UK, where they kept me in hospital for another full day after the surgery. The nose surgery was in the USA, where they seem to be desperate to get rid of you as soon as they possibly can. This is due to the way the hospitals are paid for their services and little to do with you.

Have you peed yet?

For some reason, general anesthetic can badly affect the male urogenital system. Using words I recognize, don't send a man home after surgery, until he's peed. In the UK, they kept me in hospital for 24 hours. In the US, they sat me in a recliner and bugged me every few minutes about peeing. I could only go home after performing. Until then, I could try to get comfortable in the wonderful recliner and attempt to shake off the effects of the anesthetic.

I seem to have a problem with anesthetics. I came around from one procedure to be told I'd died and they had revived me with difficulty. They suggested I used a different hospital for the MRI I was there to have. I'm claustrophobic and have had so many I can only have them when unconscious.

In the UK, they also wanted to be sure my stomach was ok and I wasn't nauseous. In the U.S., they gave me a puke bag or, as happened following several of my surgeries, an empty Wall-Mart bag. I once upchucked in one, as they wheeled me to my car. They gave me the bag with my vomit back, as soon as I was in my car. I was so grateful I kept tight hold of the bag all the way home. I lay around for the rest of the day, disappointed no one fed me grapes, but such is life. I actually don't think I'd have been able to eat the grapes, peeled or not, but it would have been nice if someone had been kind enough to ask.

Recovery

Let's go back to my second nose surgery. I'm in a recliner chair. My nose is swollen and packed on the inside with enough bandages to fill the empty space in my head. This means I must breathe through my mouth and make all those delightful noises men and women so love their spouses to make. I talk of the horrors of snoring. The outside of my nose is encased in a thin metal plate. My eyes are black and blue and my lips are swollen. I'm groggy and all I have on is one of those super sexy backless hospital gowns. Ann wants to go home and so do I; at least I think I do. I'm not sure where I am, or what's happened. It's possible I want to climb to the top of a climbing frame and do my Pavarotti impression. I do know I don't need a pee. I'm sure I won't want to pee for several days and I can't understand what peeing has to do with having my nose messed with.

Make no decisions

When you have surgery, they warn you not to sign any documents or make any life changing decisions. I can testify to this need from when I'd had my wisdom teeth removed. Ann and I were engaged and she was the dental nurse. Once I was finished, I sat in the waiting room until Ann was ready to take me home. The laughing gas had loosened my tongue and, every patient told Ann I was spilling all our secrets. My mouth was full of those cotton wool balls they pack the wounds with, so I wasn't understandable. I wanted to stop talking, but I couldn't. Many people think this problem still exists. Again, I would argue that they are wrong, although I will admit there could be a vanishingly small likelihood they are right.

I hope you can still remember the scene, me looking as if I'd lost a boxing match and I had to pee, or go back to sleep so I'd stop talking for a while. The next few hours went like this.

2:00pm
Ann "Dave, do you need to go to the bathroom?"
Dave: "No."
2:15pm
Ann: "Do you need to go to the bathroom yet?"
Dave: "Not yet."
2:30pm
Ann: "Dave, do you need to go to the bathroom?"
Dave: "No."
Ann "Can you at least try?"
Dave heads to the bathroom and sits on the toilet for several minutes.
Ann, when David returns: "Did you go?"
Dave: "No."
2:50pm
Ann (Pleading) "Do you need to go yet?"
Dave: (Who had fallen asleep.) "What? Who? What do you want?"
Ann (Pointing at the bathroom) "Bathroom?"
Dave: "Bathroom? No. I don't need to go."
Ann (Handing David a glass of water) "Then drink some water."
Dave takes a small sip of water and goes to put the glass down.

Ann: "No drink some more."

3:05pm

Ann: "Dave please go to the bathroom and try to pee."

Dave returns to the bathroom, shuts the door, rearranges the hospital gown and lowers himself onto the toilet, where he sits in a haze for some time.

Nurse- calling through the door: "Are you ok, Mr. Gray."

Dave: "Yes."

Dave shuffles back out and staggers back to the recliner

3:30pm

Ann: "Dave, toilet?"

Dave: "Nope."

3:45pm

Ann: "Dave please go to the bathroom and try."

Dave: "Ok, I'll try."

Ann "Please try hard this time"

Dave: "Ok."

4:00pm

Ann "Dave?"

Dave: "I can't and I actually feel sick."

4:05pm

A nurse puts an anti sickness drug into the IV in Dave's hand.

Dave: "Why can't I pee?"

Nurse" "It's the anesthetic drug affecting you."

Ann "How long does it normally take for them to pee?"

Nurse: "There is no set time. It can be immediately after the Surgery or it can take hours."

Ann: "It's already been 3 hours. Come on Dave, please try."

Dave again shuffles off to the bathroom and sits on the toilet, unsuccessfully willing his bladder to empty.

4:15pm

Ann "Please go to the bathroom, we need to go."

Dave returns to the bathroom but returns defeated.

04:30pm
Ann: "Dave?"
Dave goes to the bathroom again and returns triumphantly.
Dave: "I peed."
Ann jumps up and celebrates: **"Can we go home now?"**
Nurse: "He can get dressed now."
Ann helps Dave get dressed and they wait and wait and wait for the nurse to return.
05:10pm *The nurse returns with the release papers and Ann takes David home, along with his puke bag lovingly clutched to his chest.*

No eye

Returning to eye surgery and eye popping for a few minutes. We had a foster child with a glass eye. Caroline had lost her right eye at 14 months, after her mother didn't take her to the hospital when her eye needed care. The surgeons had removed her eye, to remove a tumor. Had mom gone earlier, they may have been able to save the eye. When they offered us the chance to take her into our home, we had some major decisions to make. She was our second foster placement and so we had no experience. She had a glass eye, which needed constant care and we had to learn to manage the issues with it. To remove it, you pushed under the lower lid and pushed the eye out of the socket. It made an unpleasant popping, sucking sound as it came out. We'd clean the eye and the socket then put it back.

No one believed me when I argued I could do it, not even me. I had to show my skill. That first time was hard. I'm no longer squeamish, but I was then. Like most men, I'd hoped my wife would be the responsible one and deal with eye issues. No one believed me and I had to prove I could. As Caroline wasn't coming to live with us if I didn't show I could remove and replace the eye, I chose to show them. This is how life often is. We must choose to do something unpleasant, before we can do what we wanted to do in the first place.

After the first time, it is generally easier. This is as true of what we should do, as what we shouldn't.

For me?

There are several fun stories about Caroline and her eye. The best, in my opinion, occurred in a supermarket checkout line when a woman did a thing I do a lot. That is, talk to a little person in the cart ahead of me. Occasionally, the little one doesn't want to talk. On this day, Caroline definitely didn't want to be spoken to and she showed it in the worst possible way.

The woman probably wishes she'd quit after her first failed attempt. Unfortunately, she kept trying. After a few minutes, Caroline held her hand out to the woman, who asked the obvious question, "For me?" Caroline nodded and dropped what she had into the woman's hand. The woman looked down and was totally freaked out when she saw an eye. She looked at her hand, then at Caroline who was giving an "I dare you to say anything" look. Somehow, the woman hadn't noticed the gaping hole where the eye was supposed to be. She did double takes between her hand and Caroline's zombie face. She then screamed loudly enough to be heard three counties away. Ann noticed the sound, grabbed the eye from the woman's shaking hand, and quickly put it back. It took some time to calm the woman down. I wonder if she still talks to children in shopping carts. I doubt I would if it had been me.

Don't ask her if she swallowed it!

Another time, the eye vanished and Caroline refused to say where it was. A false eye isn't too big and no easier to find than a marble. Rooms were tossed, but no eye was found. Then the worst possible thing happened. Someone asked Caroline if she'd swallowed the eye.

I know how stubborn Caroline was. With poop on her fingers and poop drawn art on the wall of her bedroom, she'd deny she did it. We had a cherry tree in our yard and I once thought she had eaten some seeds, which weren't cherries and were poisonous. She refused to answer if she had eaten any. I told her she wasn't in trouble, yet she still refused to say one way or the other. I eventually decided it wasn't worth arguing with her and simply hoped she wouldn't start vomiting.

This should have given some warning, or at least a heads up, on where the eye was or wasn't. She'd refused to say while the house had been searched. Now the horror of her having swallowed the eye was clear on the adult's faces. They did what seemed to be the only sensible thing to do.

With a solemn face, Caroline agreed she had swallowed it. A quick trip to the emergency room followed. Before x-rays or exploratory surgery was done, the ER nurse decided to take Caroline's long white socks off. Imagine the surprise and relief when, from one sock, the eye fell out from where she had hidden it next to her ankle. The only person who showed no emotion was Caroline. She didn't show anything on her face but I have to believe that she was enjoying all the problems she was causing.

Zombie

My favorite experience was when we forgot to put the eye in before we sent her out to play.

Each night, we'd take the eye out and clean it and the eye socket. In the morning, we had to clean the socket again and pop the eye back in. The amount of goop she could generate in the socket was amazing and took a few minutes to clean out. This morning we forgot to put her eye in and sent her out zombie style. She and Amy who was eight years old, visited with the widow who lived at the other end of the street. When they returned, we noticed she was missing an eye and quickly popped it in. The neighbor didn't mention it, but I wonder what she thought. The muscles were still there and the eye was designed to fit exactly on top and moved with the good eye.

Caroline was too young to do any of the other fun pranks I've heard from people with glass eyes. I'm sure she has taken the opportunity to pull them on people in the years since she left us. A glass eye that looks real, allows for many possibilities with mathematical instruments such as compasses, or with knitting needles.

Her ability to keep a straight face, showing little or no emotion will have come in useful in turning a real pain into joy, at least for her. I would not be surprised if she used it to spook other children by poking herself in the glass eye, or removing it to scare them.

What's afoot?

I had a friend at school with a prosthetic leg. He'd get into trouble from the PE teacher, when we were playing soccer. He'd loosen the straps on the leg and kick the ball. The unfortunate goalkeeper would have the sight of a ball, a foot and a leg heading for him. This memory is one that tickles my amygdala every time. My spirit bubble fills with joy and I can feel the giggles building in my stomach.

Override

The secret of happiness isn't in doing what one likes, but in liking what one does. (James M. Barrie)

I have learned how to override the pain messages battering my brain. I can't do it all the time, but those times I can are wonderful. I am acting instead of being acted upon. Pain is the body's way of telling us that there is a problem at the place that's hurting. If we stand on something sharp, the brain has learned to move our foot away from the object. If the pain continues, our brain will try one of the many alternative strategies previously used. If none works, we'd find ourselves stuck with the sharp object.

Those who don't feel pain may sound lucky. They aren't, because they can cause serious life threatening damage to their bodies. They can burn, cut and generally hurt themselves with no knowledge of the fact. They then get infections that also don't hurt, but can kill them. Pain is necessary to avoid long-term damage, but it normally goes away after the trauma is over. It doesn't for me, because whatever originally was damaged is no longer traumatized, it has repaired, but still hurts!

Broken arm

I broke my upper left arm in March 2002 and surgeons put an intermedullary rod in the following day. In English, they drilled a hole in the two bones and pushed in a rod, to make up for the two-inch gap. I asked the doctor how I lost two inches and he told me a one-ton car rolling over me would do it. The bone didn't heal, so in June 2002 they removed the rod, to see if having the loose bones rub together (a highly painful situation), would force my body to heal naturally.

All that happened was I lost my ability to use the arm. The shoulder and upper bones moved but the lower bones didn't. In November 2002, they ground up a dead woman and, using the

211

resulting putty, filled the hole on one side and put a plate on the other side. When the cast, which held my arm with the elbow bent at 90 degrees, came off in February 2003, I could use the arm. Physically the arm is fixed. I still feel the horrible pain that started at 3:04pm on March 24, 2002, near milepost 6 on Highway 25 in Colorado. The only time I've slept for more than 20 minutes, has been during the many surgeries I've undergone. Even then I didn't have a good sleep.

I was never told the identity of the woman, or how they made the putty. I apparently was one of the first people to have the procedure. One or two people have wondered about the gender of my left arm. I have to admit I don't know.

Brain confusion

My brain mishandles pain messages and causes my body to behave as if the trauma recently occurred. This usually involves vasoconstriction, narrowing or constriction of blood vessels by small muscles in their walls. When they constrict, blood flow is slowed or blocked, stopping any bleeding, but causing lots of pain.

Despite everything I've studied about the brain, all I've learned to do is override the pain messages and move them down from 10/10 to something I can manage.

My spirit is sitting in the captain's chair and, by lowering the pain gate shields, can override any pain for a brief time. Occasionally, I can get down to a 4/10 but the effort is tiring and I can't maintain the override for very long.

My life was turned over

I have mentioned the 2002 accident my family was involved in. It is a personal example of how a split-second decision can put your life on a totally different path. Mine wasn't a decision like Darius' father who was repeating an action he'd probably taken many times before. It led to him being jailed and his son left with permanent brain damage.

My decision **is** something I had done possibly millions of times before the accident and as many times since. I was overtaking a slower moving vehicle. This split-second decision changed what had been a wonderful vacation, into unbelievable horror in five horrible seconds. It was a Sunday afternoon, March 24, 2002, and my life was turned completely upside down.

The trauma from it changed my life dramatically. Traumatic is too small a word to use. Shocking, harrowing, painful, distressing are still insufficient adjectives. Sounds dramatic, I know and I can say I get pleasure from being dramatic, but can't claim to be a drama queen, as two of my daughters fulfill the role in our family. What happened though does call for dramatic adjectives.

We were on a figurative trip down the mountain with no control over what was happening, or where circumstances would lead us. At 3:05 that afternoon, we were on the second day of our trip home to Flower Mound, Texas from a vacation in Utah to have Matthew and Elizabeth sealed to us in the Salt Lake City Temple. Ann and I are Latter-day Saints, and believe a family is forever. Temples are where our marriage is sealed for time and all eternity.

We'd adopted Elizabeth and Matthew on February 20, 2002. Matthew at 9:00a.m. and Elizabeth immediately after. Until then, they weren't related to each other, but the way in which they'd come to live with us allowed us to adopt them together. Simon was attending BYU Idaho in Rexburg, Idaho and Andrew had recently left the college to prepare to serve an LDS mission.

We'd set off for the 1500-mile journey home on Saturday, March 23, Matthew's 1st birthday. By Sunday afternoon, we were at mile marker 6 on I25 in Colorado and were still only half-way home. I'd hoped to be home before 10pm, as I had to be at work in the morning and could only charge my client my outrageous fees, if I was there.

Settling down for the last 700 miles

It is 3:04pm on Sunday, March 24, 2002, and we're driving along I25, in Colorado, about 6 miles from the border with New Mexico. Ann and I are in the front of our Red 1997 Suburban. She is asleep, with the seat reclined. In the middle row are 10-year-old Elizabeth, 1-year-old Matthew and 19-year-old Andrew. 15-year-old Amy is lying

213

with her legs around 2-month-old Emily's car seat. Andrew is behind Ann, reading me a book. Elizabeth is behind me. Matthew and Emily are both asleep in their car seats. Elizabeth and Matthew had recently swapped seats to fix the perennial childhood fight over leg space, between Elizabeth and Andrew. Elizabeth has her knees up in the back of my seat watching for the New Mexico border. What happens next will change our family's life permanently and in completely different ways for each of us. None of us has any idea what is about to happen. We all assume we will make it home soon and our lives will continue the way they have.

It began at 3:05pm

At 3:05pm, the car will do something it had done many times during our trip from Dallas, Texas to Rexburg, Idaho and back. I intended to talk with the dealership about it, after we were home. The front left brake would bind on, pulling the car to the left.

This time it would be catastrophic. Another dramatic word, I know, but tragic and disastrous don't really describe what happened. At 3:04pm, the weather is sunny, the traffic is light and we are still a long way from home with 800 miles still to go. Sitting quietly, minding its own business on the left shoulder, 0.25 miles past mile marker 6, is a snow pole. It's no longer fulfilling its purpose in life. It should be standing proudly, showing where the road is, when there is several feet of snow. For some reason, it's lying on the ground sticking out about a foot into the tarmac on the left shoulder of the road. No one knows why. If it could speak, it might tell about a car that had wandered off the road and attacked it, leaving it where it now lay. It may have no memory of how it finished off where it lay. After all it was an inanimate object, so it probably doesn't. Even had it been sentient, it couldn't have known that, in a few seconds, it would play the starring role in turning the lives of all my family completely upside down, causing huge pain and setting us on a path completely different from the one we were on.

On the roof of the car are our suitcases. Everything was under a tarpaulin type of sheet, with clasps holding it to the roof rack. I was unaware the extra height had shifted the car's center of balance dangerously close to failure. I only found out that this was possible long after the accident.

We'd recently had lunch and settled down for the last part of the journey. I'd just asked Elizabeth to stop pushing against my back with her knees. In a few seconds, the brake will bind on again; pull the car to the left allowing the snow pole to cause untold problems for my family and me. The car is on cruise control, doing 70mph in, what I learned later, is a 65mph zone.

The silver pickup truck in front of me is doing 65mph, so I pull out to overtake. I'm listening to Andrew read to me, to make sure I can stay awake, as we drove through New Mexico and some of the most boring terrain on the journey. If you're from New Mexico I apologize for calling your state boring. It's nothing more than my opinion about some of the most uninteresting roads I have ever traveled. You may have found some other boring roads like along I80 in Wyoming which is slightly more interesting, in my opinion, than I40 in New Mexico.

Everything is coming together for a catastrophe

Traveling behind us is a doctor and his wife. About 100 yards ahead, traveling in the opposite direction are two ambulances full of most of the paramedics for a hundred miles. They had been scuba diving in the mountains of New Mexico. With them was the Medical Examiner. I have always been confused at where in the Raton Pass in the mountains of New Mexico they were practicing scuba diving, but have never tried to find out.

Up until 3:05pm, we'd had a wonderful vacation with our children. It had culminated in having our recently adopted children sealed to us in a ceremony at the Salt Lake City, Utah LDS temple.

We're still behind the truck when the brakes bind, pulling the steering to the left and the front left tire hits the snow pole. Somehow, the pole bounces under the car, noisily banging on the bottom. At the

215

same time as I am pulling the car back onto the road, the pole manages to exit the right side of the car and stop long enough to rip a two-foot long hole in the outer side of the front right tire.

Just five more seconds

We are five seconds from disaster, as the car's front right side rears up like a frightened animal. I manage to bring the car back down to the ground. By now, the tire has explosively deflated. The luggage and the center of balance problem, was now to play their part in the tragedy. The car veered to the right with the front right corner at a dangerously low angle. The straps holding the luggage on the roof decided now was a good time to snap, causing the car to continue sinking to the right, as the suitcases came off the roof.

Up until this moment, all of us in the car are sharing the same experience, all in a separate way. The overarching experience at the moment is we are on a journey home. What each of us is doing, though, is very different. Ann is still asleep. Andrew is reading. Matthew is dozing in his car seat. Elizabeth is poking me in the back with her knees and watching the mile-marker numbers count down to one. Amy is lying in the back seat, reading a romance novel set in Hawaii and Emily is asleep in her car seat. The only one aware that a catastrophe may be about to occur is me, as I fight to regain control of the car. Had I succeeded, we would have pulled to the edge of the road, changed the tire and been on our way again within 30 or 40 minutes laughing about the disaster we'd so narrowly avoided.

This unfortunately isn't going to happen, as it only takes a second for the car's center of gravity to move to the point of no return and the car is pulled onto its right side. Our forward motion spins it back onto its wheels and over a further four times, before coming to rest back on its wheels. We roll up an embankment then back onto I25 where we stop. Traffic begins to move slowly past us in the other lane.

Time slowed

Everything slows as the world spins round in front of me. For a couple of seconds it feels as if I am on a fairground ride. Then I black out for a short time. When I became aware of my surroundings again, we're stationary and the alarm telling me the engine is off, but the keys are in the ignition, is sounding. I turn the engine off, remove the keys and drop them to the floor.

For a few seconds, I can't work out what had happened and then... Matthew is screaming. Ann is sitting up and bleeding badly from her head. The front roof console is broken and hanging down above her. The windshield is shattered, as is the driver's door window.

I look at Ann and ask, "What happened?"

"Burst tire." She replied.

My left arm is in pain and I turn to my left to see what's wrong. At the same time, a man who identifies himself as the county coroner appears at my side and asks if I am Ok. My arm is hanging out of the broken window. It's broken and the lower arm is hanging the wrong way. When I look out the window, my left hand is pointing at a body lying on the ground, next to the rear door. Even though the body is covered, I know it's Elizabeth. I can see her red hair. Andrew and Amy are also missing. I look around and see them lying some 150 yards away, on Ann's side of the car. The children are surrounded by people. I tell the coroner I'm not sure how I feel.

Different points of view

There are many points of view about the effect of those 5 seconds. The paramedics had to deal with the emotional and mental pain from chasing Andrew and Amy as they bounced, at high-speed, along the highway. Once they caught up with the children, they did their jobs. I can't see how Andrew or Amy would have survived without them,

The doctor ran up to Amy and started to deal with the fact that her lungs had collapsed by intubating her. His wife got Matthew out and calmed him down. The driver of the truck saw I'd lost control and accelerated out of the way, then reversed back to help.

These people have all had to deal with the pain of being involved in what happened that day. I've no idea how they've handled their pain in the years since, but I'm confident it had some effect. An accident with bodies all over the road is hard to forget.

Those of us in the car suffered directly from the crash, but all in different ways. Our injuries were completely different. The list is long and horrible including broken necks, backs, arms, hands, pelvis', hips, feet, jaws, skulls, elbows, lungs, spleens etc., etc. Some of us suffered all of them, some a few, one suffered none. I was left disabled and in chronic pain.

The pain wasn't only physical; it was mental, spiritual and emotional as well. It still bothers us. It isn't an every day, all day type of issue, it is more that a scab has formed over the hurt. We would be insane to pick at that scab.

Getting home again

We filled the ICU unit for two nights and the operating theaters for the next 10 days, as the doctors kept finding parts to stitch back together.

Amy kept fading in and out of a coma and, at least four or five times a day for the first week, we had to convince her we'd had an accident. First, we were in Colorado not Hawaii. She thought she was in the novel she'd been reading, which was set in Hawaii. Her bed was facing a window with a view of a wall of the hospital. We couldn't be in Colorado, because there were no mountains. We also had to convince her something that was a lot harder on us. We had to convince Amy that Elizabeth was dead.

The spiritual and emotional pain of trying to convince her of a horrible fact we didn't want to believe ourselves was difficult. The fact Elizabeth was in a fridge somewhere, we didn't even know where, was hard enough. Having to repeat what had happened and tell Amy that

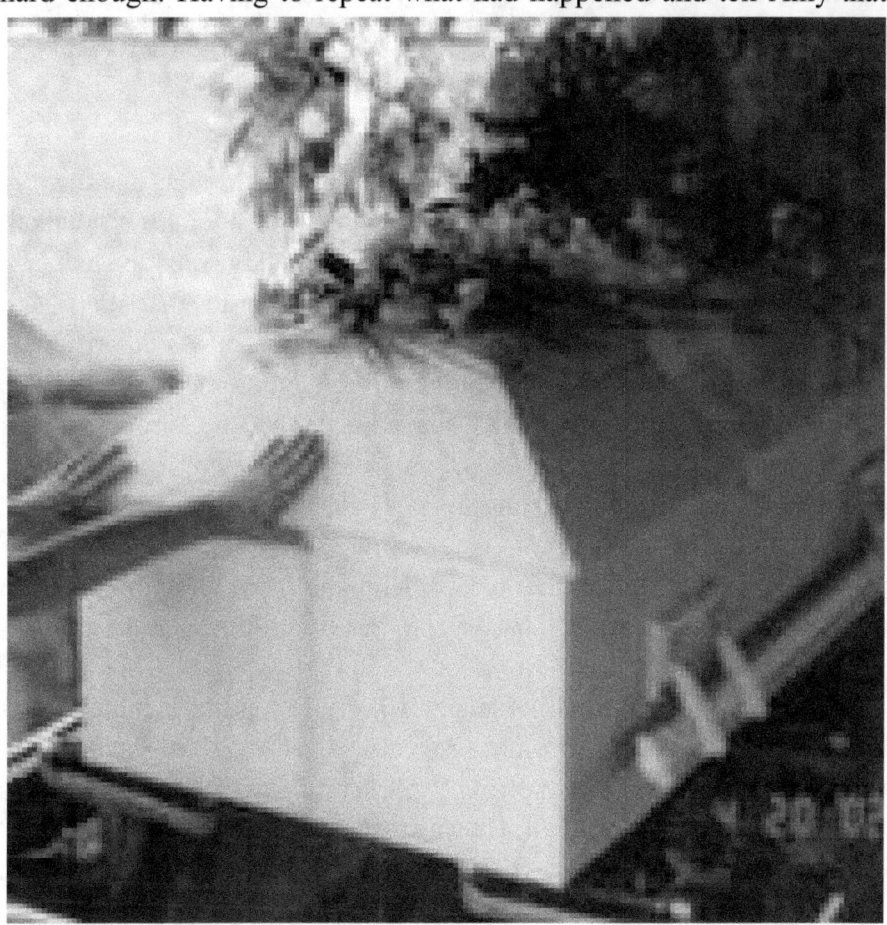

Elizabeth had died in the accident, every few hours, was difficult for me to have to do. I had no choice; it wasn't her fault she couldn't remember. This is one memory in which I can find no joy; I cannot turn the experience into one where there can be humor.

Burying our daughter

Amy and I were the last to return home, on April 16. No one had fully recovered, but at least we were home, 24 days after setting off.

We buried Elizabeth nearly four weeks after the accident on Saturday, April 20, 2002. The date was odd in that we had adopted her and Matthew on February 20th, 2002. On March 20th, 2002, we had them sealed to us in the Salt Lake City LDS temple in Salt Lake City, Utah. Somehow, here we were on April 20, burying her in a cemetery in Flower Mound Texas.

You're movie extras, aren't you?

We looked as if we were extras from a movie. In fact, one night in Walt-Mart, an associate asked if we were. The TV show, Walker, Texas Ranger was filmed nearby and she assumed we must be extras.

A terrible assumption, but clearly possible to the Wall-Mart associate this evening. I'd had my hair cut short to show solidarity with Ann. My left arm was in a sling and I had some road rash injuries.

Ann's head had been totally shaved, to allow the surgeons to fix her scalp and skull. She had splints on both hands and, most obvious, she had a horrendous looking metal halo screwed into her skull, supporting her broken neck.

Simon hadn't been in the accident, but had come home from college. He has cerebral palsy and, at that time, was using his wheelchair.

Andrew was showing evidence of horrible road rash injuries. His right arm was in a sling from a broken collarbone, which occurred in the hospital, and he was wearing a back brace as he had broken his hips and back in the accident. He was using crutches.

Amy also had a strange hairstyle from the multiple surgeries on her skull and face. She had many road rash injuries, a broken skull, broken face and a full body cast from a broken back, hips and pelvis. The body cast was reminiscent of the armor Xena, Warrior Princess, wore. She was also on crutches.

We were the walking wounded, not unlike people who had been involved in a nasty car accident. Which we had. The Wall-Mart associate refused to believe we weren't acting and only left us alone, when I showed her the pictures of Elizabeth's funeral I'd just picked up from the photo lab.

None of us looked good for several months after, but eventually, the most obvious physical deficits went away.

Accepting it is what it is

Finding peace is the primary way to become happy and produce endorphins. For me, that peace is related to acceptance of what is. I still have moments where it's all too much for me to handle. So far, I've always found a way back, by looking for and finding joy and happiness. I have found and used tried and tested methods of positively charging my spirit bubble. The accident happened and I can change nothing about it. Absolutely nothing. What has happened cannot be undone or modified to fit what I wanted.

This is true for everyone involved. Our points of view are all totally different on what happened and the effect they had on each of us.

Yet each of us has had to come to terms with it and accept that it is what it is and rebuild our lives from that point forward. Elizabeth's death is also something that affected us all differently. Ann and I lost a daughter, Simon, Andrew, Amy and Matthew lost a sister. Emily lost a sister too, but at that point in time, Elizabeth was her foster sister. We had yet to adopt Emily at that point.

Parental Grief

As most people tend to die from old age, parents aren't supposed to die before their children do, so it is a difficult concept to understand.

In her book, Surviving Grief. Catherine M Sanders writes ***"The reason parental grief is so different from other losses has to do with excess. Because loss of a child is such an unthinkable loss, everything is intensified, exaggerated and lengthened. Guilt and anger are usually present in every significant loss, but these emotions are inordinate with grieving parents. Experts estimate it takes anywhere from three to five years to reach renewal after a*** *spouse dies, but parental grief might go on for ten to twenty years or maybe a lifetime."*

We didn't take that long, although there's a hole where Elizabeth is supposed to be even now. I spent months, working with a therapist, to get from the point where, every time I thought about the pain in my arm, I saw my daughter's dead body below my hand. This is when I moved from having victim mentality, to being a victim of an event that occurred in the past. I want her to be here, but she isn't and life has to go on with or without her. I still mourn her many years later but there is nothing I can do to bring her back.

Grief

Grief is one of the hardest parts of having RSD. Ann and I have come to terms with Elizabeth's death. What RSD has taken from me has been as hard to come to terms with.

Most experts say there are five stages of grief.

1. Denial and Isolation
2. Anger
3. Bargaining
4. Depression
5. Acceptance

Using the order above, the first reaction to a major trauma such as the death of a loved one, is to deny anything happened. This defense mechanism buffers us from the immediate shock. We block out the words and hide from reality. This temporary response carries us through the first wave of pain.

Next is anger, which may be aimed at inanimate objects, complete strangers, friends or family. We may be angry with our deceased loved one. Rationally, we know the person isn't at fault. Emotionally, however, we may resent the person for causing us pain, or for leaving us. We feel guilty for being angry, and this makes us angrier. I went through this.

After anger, we may find ourselves bargaining to regain control, and begin to wonder if we could undo what has happened.

Depression is a reaction to loss. Sadness and regret are common in this type of depression. We worry about the costs of burial. We worry that, in our grief, we've spent less time with those who depend on us. We worry about the way we look, because we cry so much or because we are worrying too much.

Acceptance is the one stage generally last. This is where we accept what has happened and we calm down, or become as calm as we were before or we can be. This stage can be the longest, especially when the trauma such as the death of a family member or a chronic pain which doesn't go away. Eventually, we accept it, or go mad.

What if the problem can't be solved?

Sometimes the storms we are suffering through are problematical. Some don't seem to be solvable, no matter what we try or how hard we try. Right now, I have a boatload of problems to resolve. At the same time, none of the problems I was suffering with last week have gone away and some have got worse. I must somehow resolve them all, but I have no idea how to do this! Some are problems caused by lack of money or what money is being spent on. This is the number one issue that breaks up many marriages.

So, if we can't sort problems out, what can we do? One thing is worry. From personal experience, I know how worrying makes everything worse, because it fills my spirit bubble with negative emotions. I've suffered too many nights worrying about things and succeeded in nothing more than being tired the next day. I was also a lot crankier than I normally was, never a good idea no matter who you are.

Don't worry, <u>do</u> what you <u>can</u>.

I recently watched as two small birds chased off a large crow. I assume they were worried about it and didn't trust it wouldn't attack their nest. What they didn't do is sit there and squawk about the fact there were crows, they did something about it. They chased it away and it then

223

found itself under attack from another set of birds, even smaller than the first pair. The small birds could have simply worried about the crow and done nothing. They decided to do what they could, knowing they may have come off second best. Even though there **are** things we need to be concerned about, many of them never happen. Those that do, happen in a way we can generally manage.

For example, we go to the person from whom we borrowed $300 and we have no money to pay them back. Before we even have a chance to explain, they tell us they have a payment plan and we can pay it off with a deposit of $25. As long as the whole amount is paid within the next two months all is well.

We'd spent the night worrying, getting no sleep and then were unpleasant to our family for no reason. We should have spent the night not worrying and telling ourselves we would ask for some sort of payment plan, then not worry about what to do if they deny our request. We would have been much happier.

This is where we can take charge; where we can act instead of being acted upon. We can remind ourselves of the many times the thing we've been worrying about has happened in the horrendous way we had imagined; which generally has been zero.

What is the worst that can happen?

Ask what is the worst that can happen. I have tried this myself many times and have found I can handle even the worst scenario. I have constantly tried it with my children. I have reminded them so far that none of their worst fears has been realized. Even when they did; they had the ability to handle it. If the worst that can happen is to leave us where we are, why are we wasting time, energy and emotional strength worrying about it?

While I was chaperoning at a dance, one of my children wanted to go ask a girl to dance. I asked him the question, what is the worst that can happen? They wouldn't be dancing with her. This is where he was now and would be the worst that could happen. So, quit worrying what she might say and ask her, or stop bugging me. Of course, I had the same worries when I was a teenager. Maybe learning that we shouldn't worry about things we have no control over, is part of growing up.

One unbelievably sad and weird news story told about a young man killing his father. He killed him in an argument over whether the father was safe, while in the shower with the front door unlocked. This is taking worrying to its ultimate destructibility. Singer Carrie Underwood suggests in her song, the way to get past our worries is to have Jesus take the wheel,

Facebook is not the answer either

These Facebook posts from my 14-year-old daughter say it all.

For all those teens complaining about not getting sleep... Instead of browsing Facebook, Instagram, Tumblr, YouTube, Netflix, etc. For 7 hours or more. Why don't you try putting your phone down? Let the phone charge without you playing on it. It's bad for the battery if you're on it while it's charging. That or consider seeing a doctor and see if you have insomnia.

......

Nothing personal about my recent post, but it gets annoying because I just see posts about not getting enough sleep. Also, posting your issues on Facebook won't solve your problems. Again, no shade to those of you who post about not sleeping.

Don't worry – be happy

There are times when we must worry, like how do I pay the funeral costs for my dead daughter. This needed resolving but doing nothing except worrying will change nothing. We must do what we can to resolve or improve the situation. When there's nothing more we can do, we need to accept things are what they are. We can then get on with our lives, the best we can. Obviously I couldn't just ignore the problem of Elizabeth's funeral expenses. I had to do what I could to find the money. It was no use just worrying, because that would not have provided me with a loan, or donation to a fund, or whatever I could come up with doing. I had to decide if this was the worst that could happen and whether it was acceptable to me. I didn't need to worry they'd dig Elizabeth back up and deliver her and her coffin to my house, because that is illegal. The worst would be having to sell something or go begging. For many of us, having to ask for help can be the worst thing that could happen and be totally unacceptable.

A friend was staring at the horror of a prison sentence. His future was in the hands of the judge. To his credit, my friend spent the time between his guilty plea and sentencing, doing everything he could to live normally. He still went to jail, but he didn't make the problem worse by putting himself in jail for the previous 6 months with none stop worrying.

Leaving them behind and having to move on

Ann and I have gone through the grief steps many times, as our foster children have left us. To us, it has been the same as if they'd died, because we never see them again.

Selena is one of our foster children we had to leave behind and this wasn't a choice we made voluntarily or willingly. We'd one spare seat in our car when we headed to Idaho in 2002 and wanted to take her with us. Her social worker was one of those soulless, heartless witches we've occasionally worked with. We also had Selena's sister, Skyla and for some reason, she didn't want to let us to take Selena with us. She'd allow us to take Skyla, in fact, she insisted we do so, but we weren't having our own way. We didn't want to take Skyla, as she had problems that would make the journey impossible.

We had taken Selena on the same journey the year before. As we wouldn't do as the social worker demanded, both girls were sent to a respite foster home for the two weeks we were supposed to be away. When those two weeks turned into six weeks, because we had a car wreck, they stayed at the respite home. The worker then made sure we couldn't take either girl back. I don't know why she did this and she is one of the few people I really don't like.

No amount of training prepared us for the horror of losing Selena at the same time as losing Elizabeth. The fact Selena isn't dead, doesn't make the loss any easier. We learned the hard way how everything can go wrong, because of the actions of people we thought were on our side. With Selena, we finished off being the victims and a social worker was the perpetrator of the abuse.

Worrying about the problem was of no use to Selena or us. We could have lain in bed trying to solve the problem and succeeded in doing nothing more than making our issues with sleeping even worse.

Selena's father did eventually finish off paying for some of his actions. The original judge's decision made him believe he could get away with anything. His behavior eventually crossed the line and the police were called to arrest him. His arrogance meant he was hog-tied and carried out of the CPS office into the police car. I never found out what happened to him, but I hope he was made to pay for the horror he put his wife and children through for 10+ years. He should serve nothing less, in my admittedly judgmental opinion.

Look, a baby!

We had a lot of fun with Selena. The first time she didn't have the same worker as when she came back. She was with us when we drove from Texas to Idaho to see our son Andrew, during BYU Idaho's Mother's Week. Selena was an instant hit. We attended a meeting in one of the conference centers on campus and took Selena with us.

The main speaker commented that typically when he was talking with a family audience, a child will stand up and in a loud voice ask, "Are we finished yet?" He remarked he didn't expect this to happen today, as there were no children in the audience. Then he noticed Ann and Selena. He apologized and asked Ann to bring the baby up for all to see. For the rest of our time on campus, Selena was a star and everyone wanted to meet her.

These memories and some pictures are all we have to remember her, but they are all happy memories.

Our children have all suffered through the grief stages with something unbelievably hard. They've lost their parents. We all eventually must go through this loss, but our children have lost their parents, even though they're still alive. As well as being confusing, this loss is hard to deal with when you're young. I know losing a parent is hard to deal with when you are an adult. I simply cannot comprehend how it feels when you're only little.

Celiac's disease

With RSD and Celiac's disease, the grief and loss can be as hard as it is to lose a loved one. My grandparents, father, a daughter, both parents in law, a niece and a nephew have all passed on. Over 120 foster children no longer live with us and we suffered through a death in utero. I believe I understand the grief of losing loved ones. This is how I can say RSD and Celiac disease bring with them a loss and associated grief.

With Celiac disease, denial is hard once you have a diagnosis, because Montezuma's revenge follows swiftly if we eat gluten. Diagnosis began for me with an annual physical and a blood test, showing my liver numbers elevated over 1000%. I was sent for a doctor's favorite diagnosis – tests. I had another sonogram, this time over all my internal organs.

Blood tests were next and they took 35 vials of blood for various tests they needed to do. The only time I've had more blood taken was when I came second for a bone marrow donation to a child with leukemia and I lost count of the vials they filled. The other donor turned out to be an even closer match and I didn't find how painful it is to have a hole made in my hip, to help the little girl. I suppose I am happy about that because the pain from having the hole made would still be here.

You want to put it where?

Next, I had an upper endoscopy. If you've had one, you'll know how much fun they are. There are two types of endoscopy, one designed for either end of the alimentary canal. For those of us who flunked biology, or spent the time chatting up the good-looking girls, or being that girl, the alimentary canal starts at the mouth and ends at our bottom, through the esophagus, the stomach, intestines and through to the rectum.

If they want to look at the lower end of our alimentary canal, they send the camera up from the bottom end. This is done by a type of doctor that intrigues me anyone wants to become, a proctologist. There are many jokes about this profession, most of which would get me into trouble. My favorites are ***Proctologist: A brain surgeon for lawyers.*** My son-in-law is a lawyer, so this one amuses me the most. The second is supposed to have been asked a proctologist, ***"Could you write me a note for my wife, saying my head isn't, in fact, up there?"***

My proctologist introduced the camera into the spot where the sun doesn't shine and ignored me until he removed the camera. He spent the time chatting with the nurse about his recent vacation.

If they want to look at the top end of our alimentary canal, the camera goes up the nose, down the throat and into the stomach.

As I'd previously undergone both types and didn't enjoy either, I was happy to find I would be sedated. When I came to, there was a color photo on which was written **"ulcerative colitis"** lying on my chest. A few days later, 23/12 of all days, I got a phone call telling me I had Celiac disease. I say of all days not because Christmas was close, it was also the same day a few years earlier I'd broken my ankle. For the next few months, I ate a gluten free diet and had more blood tests done. This time, my numbers were all normal.

No more gluten for me.

Now I must avoid all gluten or I get sick quickly. I must have had the disease all my life, as I had the symptoms from childhood.

I have a major loss now. I can't eat my favorite pizzas; I loved 12-inch subway sandwiches, but can no longer eat anything made with wheat bread. I must eat bread 1/4 to 1/2 the size of wheat bread, in a loaf 1/3rd the size, for 4 times the cost. Each slice also has twice the calories of its bigger brother.

I can't eat at fast food restaurants, because the food has wheat, or has been contaminated. Even burgers have flour! If I make my children a sandwich, I must remember to wash my hands. I must check the labels of everything I eat, as even chocolate may have wheat.

I grieve for what was, what might have been, what never will be again. In this case, the mental pain of not being able to eat what I want. The emotional pain of not easily finding what I can eat then not enjoying eating it. I mourn my loss not quite as badly as with the death of a loved one and have the same stages of grief to go through.

I also mourn that the food I can eat, has twice the calories for half the serving and little of the taste. Before I got Celiac's disease, I had lost a lot of weight. I put it all back on again and I grieve over this.

RSD Loss

With RSD, what I have lost is different, but as much of a loss. This time, relating to physical ability. If it hurts doing what we're used to doing, the normal response is to stop doing it until it stops hurting. For example, if picking our nose with our index finger is painful, use another finger, or stop picking our nose until the finger stops hurting.

RSD means everything I want to do is difficult, or even impossible, to do without pain. As nose picking is a thing we all do, but all deny, I won't say whether I can do it without pain. What I can say is that I suffer pain when walking, running, sitting, lying down, standing up, kneeling, playing with my children and many other activities. I'm denied sleep, the ability to work and support my family and the ability to do anything without pain. I'm even denied pity parties, because most people are sick of hearing me complain.

With RSD, denial starts with the fact the condition changes my life forever. I want the doctors to be wrong about it. I want the diagnosis to be wrong and the pain to go.

The anger can be at anything. For me it's an inanimate object – the snow pole we hit. I can be angry with the doctors, who can't provide me with medication to get rid of the pain and allow me to have some sort of life. Anger is dangerous because it causes stress, depression and bitterness. Stress, by itself, causes depression, which in turn causes stress, and we're then angry. When we are grieving for what was lost, we tend to be stressed and angry. They all seem to go together in a very vicious circle.

For me, stress makes me hurt more, I feel the pain at a higher level. This causes me to become stressed and angry and around and around we go. I do my utmost to get off this merry-go-round and avoid my spirit bubble filling with negative thoughts and feelings. If I don't, I will finish off permanently angry, stressed and suffering with a lot of pain.

Critical censor

When we're stressed and angry, the chances are high that we'll say or do something we'll regret. The critical censor is the part of the limbic system tasked with censoring what we say. This is a part of the brain with a name that does what its name implies. It makes sure we don't say or do the wrong thing to the wrong person at the wrong time, or any combination of wrongness. There are two ways to turn the censor off. Alcohol is one and stress the other. As many people drink too much when they are stressed, the two often go together.

The likelihood of unpleasant behavior and shouting is much higher when the censor is switched off. When it's turned on again and we remember what we did, we find ourselves suffering mental anguish because we shouted or were rude and unpleasant. Often these go together, so we have several things to fix. We then have things to worry over and have to sort that spiral out as well. This is a slightly different sort of worry; not over what should I do, but what can I do about what I did.

Acceptance of what is.

I have accepted I have RSD and the mental anguish is almost gone. The physical problems stay, even though they're not visible. I've seen proof they exist with procedures such as nuclear medicine. Most of my problems, I can't ignore. I have no choice over walking, sitting, standing, etc. and must find a way to do so within a level of pain I can manage. If I offend people when I am stressed because of the pain level or because of the way someone else has reacted to me, I have to find a way to apologize and make them realize it is the pain doing the talking.

What do I do? How do I manage the pain, when I can't keep the pain gates blocked? I do whatever is needed to produce the feel-good brain neurotransmitters dopamine, serotonin and endorphins.

Feel Good Neuro Transmitters

In all of living have much of fun and laughter. Life is to be enjoyed, not just endured. (Gordon B. Hinckley

Before I go any further, for you who know neurology, I accept I'm about to over simplify. Imagine there are reservoirs in our brains controlling our supply of the neurotransmitters dopamine, endorphins and serotonin. Our body creates and stores them until they are needed. When needed, the valve is turned and lets the neurotransmitters flow out. Problems can and do occur when the amount we need is less than is available in the reservoir. In this case, the neurotransmitter may pass straight through without being stored in the reservoir, assuming we can manufacture more.

Producing endorphins

We'll start with endorphins, which apparently are endogenous opioid inhibitory neuropeptides. I'm none the wiser. Inhibitory I understand. Inhibit means to slow down, hold back, hinder or hamper.

A more helpful definition is that endorphins stop the transmission of pain signals and can produce euphoria, another fancy term, defined as a mental and emotional condition in which a person experiences intense feelings of well-being, elation, happiness, excitement and joy.

I want lots of endorphins please. The best endorphin producers are chocolate and ice cream. Too much of both, perversely, is bad for us, because fats can deplete us of endorphins. Dark chocolate is best for pain inhibition and, of course, I dislike dark chocolate. Good fats, from fish, nuts and fruits are the best, but they're not as good as chocolate.

In fact nothing is better than chocolate even if it has melted in the sun and is an amorphous blob.

Exercise

I'm limited in using the quickest and most powerful method of getting endorphins, exercise. Having broken my ankle, I can no longer run, even walking hurts. Poor me, I have a reason not to exercise. I used to have to come up with excuses not to exercise; now I have a good reason. The things is, 20 or more minutes of exercise releases massive amounts of endorphins and helps mask pain. I may not be able exercise much, but I can keep moving. My family constantly asks me why I don't stop and this is why. Even if I can't exercise, that doesn't mean I should become a couch potato. My medications all cause me problems with weight gain, so if I did nothing I imagine I'd be more of a blob than I already am.

Begorphins

I'm trying to produce endorphins. If I stop, I seem to get negative endorphins, we'll call them begorphins. They suck the life out of me and I sit zoned out for a while. The pain messages flood into the control room and my spirit bubble is overwhelmed with all the negativity unmanaged pain brings with it. I have to find a way to force the positivity back into my spirit bubble. I need endorphins.

How to smile and be happy

One thing that generates endorphins, which embarrass my children, especially my daughters, is to force myself to be happy. I'll talk to strangers and tell them to be happy, simply to see them smile. Their smiles make me happy. This embarrasses my daughters and this makes me happy as well. Forcing ourselves to smile makes our spirit push the *release endorphins* button. This button works in the same way as on a computer with a greyed out *continue* button. Only after we click on the agree button, accepting the terms and conditions, does the continue button become active. On a side note, great care should be taken when reading these terms and conditions. The Apple ITunes

EULA (End User Licensing Agreement) has us agree not to use ITunes to create missiles and biological, chemical, or nuclear weapons.

A company called PC Pitstop once had a clause in its EULA saying if someone read the full agreement and contacted the company, they'd receive $1000. It took 4 months before someone bothered to read the whole agreement and claim the money.

A video retailer named GameStation had a clause giving the company "a non-transferable option by which they claimed our immortal soul for now and ever more". The company took a few dollars off their next sale to anyone who demanded their soul back.

The release endorphin button doesn't need us to sell our immortal soul, to become active. Imagine the button is on the main keyboard in your control room; have your spirit press it and you will release endorphins.

I recall pleasurable activities and moments because they push the *release endorphins* button. Studies have shown that 8 to 10 minutes of laughing aloud, will create an extended elevation of endorphins, which can contribute to a better night's sleep. Be warned, those around us may worry about our mental state, 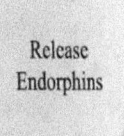 especially if we do this for 8 to 10 continuous minutes, when there is nothing they perceive as funny. I say we should ignore them!

How to generate begorphins

There are several ways to generate begorphins (the opposite of endorphins) and they are often to do with other people's unthinking attitude towards us and our problems. In most cases, they don't mean to upset, they usually succeed, though.

One top begorphins producers for me is the idea and question of, "if you could do it yesterday, (whatever "it" happens to be), how come you can't today?" This is, without doubt, the most irritating, annoying and depressing question chronic pain sufferers ever hear. Morning comes around and I get up, tireder than when I came to bed. I hurt over my whole body, but start the day as everyone else does, by staggering into the bathroom.

On a normal, average day, I'll range from 20% to 40% of how I was before I contracted RSD. In the morning, I start at 5% and get better as the day goes on. Today, I manage to get up to 50% using a combination of will power and necessity. I must pay for this extra effort the next day and so the maximum is 30%. People, who don't suffer from chronic pain, don't understand this concept and assume... I don't know what they assume. I know they give me a tough time over it. They do this, even though they understand the concept, from when they over exercise and their muscles hurt.

It seems to be easier for them, not for us, for them, to believe we are malingering. They don't want to face the truth and in some cases, especially when the sufferer is a minor, refuse to get the pain medication. They then blame us, the person with chronic pain, for making their lives harder.

For whatever reason their spirit bubbles are negatively charged and we are the supposed cause and unless we try hard our spirit bubbles will be overwhelmed. This is another situation where we act. We don't allow others to overwhelm or act on our positivity. This is an example of a big begorphin producer that is quite common, especially in families where there is someone suffering with physical, whether hidden or not, spiritual, emotional or mental pain.

A number of chronic physical pain sufferers have told me how there are days when everyone seems to be on their case and in some way attacking them. There are some days when it feels that if their body isn't giving them grief in the areas they have suffered trauma, everybody they come across, family or otherwise, is telling them they are wrong about everything and anything. They're told they are grumpy old men or women and an unpleasant [whatever role they play]. They feel they're given no leeway for the pain they're suffering and everything they say is unacceptable. If there's an insignificantly small chance that what they said could have been said in some way maliciously, they're accused of saying it with malicious intent.

Everything they do is also unacceptable even when whatever they suggested is then done by the person who told them thy were wrong.

This example is played out in many homes, in many families. In some cases one person is responsible for all the negativity and fills every family member's spirit bubble with their negativity. I could list many more begorphins, but there's not really any point because all it does is upset me.

So, …. what …

The principle of so, … what…? comes in here. **So**, others are causing us to produce begorphins, or we ourselves are being negative, **what** do I do about it? **So,** I don't like begorphins, **what** can I do to produce endorphins? We'll answer that question as we look at dopamine and serotonin.

Producing dopamine

The neurotransmitter dopamine is involved in pleasurable reward, movement, memory, attention, mood and sleep. There are several problems caused by having too little dopamine in the brain, including lack of interest in life, decreased motivation, inability to feel pleasure, altered sleep patterns, restless leg syndrome, mood swings, poor memory, inability to focus/impaired concentration and impulsive or self-destructive behaviors. The symptoms are the same as the ones for lack of sleep. They are all symptoms I suffer from. Increasing dopamine can make these symptoms improve. I can only speak for myself, but I can't get rid of the symptoms totally.

The way we interact with others is also closely related to dopamine transmission. Talking with others increases dopamine levels. Listening to others does as well. Giving service to those worse off than we are, as well as some who are better off, increases dopamine.

A quick and easy way to release dopamine is with goals. Make a list of what we want to achieve today and check them off as we do them. This releases both dopamine and endorphins and puts the pleasure center in the brain into party mode. If we get to work on time or get our degree, we'll release dopamine. Even setting a goal of not checking Facebook today and staying away from the computer is a success and our brains release dopamine. If we set goals for everything we must do, including silly items such as cleaning our teeth, and tell ourselves how well we did, the button is pressed.

Producing serotonin

The neurotransmitter serotonin helps us keep calm. It regulates moods and helps lower stress, panic and anxiety. Then there are the Selective Serotonin Re-uptake Inhibitors (SSRI) type medications such as Zoloft, Prozac and Paxil, which increase the level of serotonin by blocking its absorption. Many anti-depressants have the useful side effect of pain relief. It isn't all positive, though, as the main side effect of the ones I take, is serious weight gain. Oh well, I have to balance the relief from the pain with the horror of gaining the pounds. I'd rather not have to, but I will suffer being heavier

Release Serotonin

Eat right

To make dopamine, our bodies need to produce an amino acid called tyrosine.

We do some manufacturing, some synthesizing and some other fancy sounding terms, and at the end, we have our feel-good fuel. I'm not going to make diet suggestions other than the following simple lists.

These foods are tyrosine producers.

* Almonds,	* Bananas,
* Low-fat yogurt,	* Meat,
* Poultry,	* Avocados,
* Lima beans,	* Sesame seeds,
* Pumpkin seeds,	* Soy products.

238

These next foods increase tryptophan, which our bodies uses to create serotonin.

* Chocolate,
* Yogurt,
* Poultry, in particular chicken and turkey,
* Red meat especially beef and pork,
* Bananas,
* Citrus fruits
* Oats,
* Cottage Cheese,
* Peanuts
* Milk
* Eggs
* Vegetables,
* Fish especially salmon and tuna where omega 3 fatty acid is high,

Exercise

Exercise rears its ugly head here again by increasing blood calcium, which stimulates dopamine release and uptake in our brains. 30 to 60 minutes of walking, swimming or jogging will jump-start our dopamine and endorphin levels. Of the three, jogging and swimming hurt, so I must walk. I'm limited, but not totally incapable. **So**, it hurts to jog and swim, **what** can I do? Walk!

Laughing is good for dopamine release and uptake and it releases endorphins. An endorphin high is useful to me, because endorphins inhibit pain. Wow, a side effect of laughing, is stopping pain.

I was trying to send a text to my daughter, Angelina, recently. The predictive text and voice program couldn't understand the word "start". The text I sent said, "What time do you stop call stops Dopp begin?" The insanity made me giggle and laugh for several minutes. I had felt down and depressed up until then.

Exercise is the answer to building the neurotransmitters that help us feel well, improving our mood and producing endorphins. Sunlight is also good for us. Obviously, exercising in the sun, eating zero calorie chocolate and ice-cream, would be the best option.

Water

Whenever my family tells me they're unwell, have a headache or are in a bad mood, the first thing I ask them is, if they have drunk

239

recently. It's almost a mantra, Drink! I feel better having drunk a glass of water. Many times, we will mistake hunger for thirst and eat instead of drink. A glass of water will often stop the hunger pangs.

The experts even manage to come up with a meaningless definition for water. Here is the Wikipedia offering.

"Water (H^20) is a polar inorganic compound that is at room temperature a tasteless and odorless liquid, nearly colorless with a hint of blue. This simplest hydrogen chalcogenide is by far the most studied chemical compound and is described as the "universal solvent" for its ability to dissolve many substances. This allows it to be the "solvent of life". It is the only common substance to exist as a solid, liquid, and gas in normal terrestrial conditions."

The experts on water prove they're drips under pressure, because no two seem to be able to agree on the amount we should drink. They all seem to agree at least 44 ounces of non-caffeine, non-soda fluids is the minimum. There is a lot of research showing levels of depression decrease after a few days of drinking enough water.

I want to drink caffeinated soda, which fails on two levels. First caffeine is a diuretic, causing us to need to go to the bathroom more often and become dehydrated, which makes us depressed. Caffeine keeps us awake and inhibits serotonin levels, causing us to be depressed and irritable. Soda has a lot of sugar, as does most candy. Refined sugars cause an immediate high, which unfortunately only lasts a brief time. We then suffer a crash that leaves us tired and depressed, feeling worse than before we drank the soda or ate the candy.

You'll agree it should be otherwise, but it isn't. We'll have a pity party together right now, about how anything tasting good is generally illegal, immoral and fattening. Don't sulk for too long, there's nothing we can do about it. But, if you do find a solution, please let me know.

If not soda, then what? The simple answer is water. Drinking up to 64 fluid ounces of water a day is recommended by doctors,

Deep Breathing

We all need to breathe. No one can stop breathing for more than a few minutes without causing irreparable damage or death.

With pain and stress management, deep breathing is a method of relaxation. Pain is worse when we're stressed, so if we were relaxed, we'd feel less pain. I know how much, because I am in more pain if I am stressed; the higher the stress level the higher the pain I'm suffering. If I'm not feeling stressed; my pain levels drop. It involves using the diaphragm, a large muscle resting across the bottom of the ribs. When we breathe in, the diaphragm drops, opening space so air can come into our lungs. I use a method I call 357. Breathe in through your nose for 3 seconds, hold your breath for 5 seconds and breathe out for 7 seconds through your mouth. Try it, you may even be able to feel better about everything being illegal, immoral or fattening. I can't guarantee it will help with liking spinach or broccoli. You're aware the difference between boogers and broccoli is you can't get your children to eat broccoli.

Relax

When we breathe deeply, we activate the brain parts controlling relaxation, including the frontal lobes and the limbic system, which includes the amygdala. It also lowers our heart rate and blood pressure, decreases muscle tension and calms us. At least this is the medical description. I'm looking at finding joy while fighting the pain, so I will argue that breathing deeply will positively charge our spirit bubble and make us feel better.

Sleep

Virtually every book on the topic of managing pain says to make sure we're getting 6 to 8 hours sleep every night and aren't being disturbed while asleep. Not being able to go into a deep sleep can seriously affect our mental ability throughout the next day. My response is "You think? Thanks for the heads up."

I haven't slept for more than 20 minutes at a time, since the accident in 2002. The only times I've been unconscious for longer, is when I've been undergoing surgery. This, however, doesn't count as good sleep. I've tried sleeping tablets of all kinds, with no success.

Did you know the most common side effect of sleeping tablets is insomnia? If you think about it, this must be the most useless side effects for anything. There we are, having difficulty getting to sleep, or staying asleep, and the doctor prescribes a sleep aid, which gives us insomnia. If you haven't suffered from this problem, I can tell you it's no fun and I don't recommend you try.

I once had five days of insomnia and by the fifth day, I was seeing things. I knew they weren't real, so they didn't scare me, but it was strange. Fortunately, the following day the drugs had flushed out of my system and I returned to my earlier inability to stay asleep. I also stopped seeing things. This weird side effect problem is common, anti-depressants can cause depression; pain medication can make the pain worse. Makes you wonder if there is a conspiracy. We take a medication, but it has a side effect for which we take another medication. This second one has another unpleasant side effect, so we take another medication. If we're not careful, we'll end up taking the original medication to overcome the side effect of the earlier medication in the chain.

Serotonin is the brain chemical regulating the sleep/wake cycle. It helps us stay asleep when we should be and awake when we should be. When serotonin levels aren't normal, sleep disturbances, depression and chronic fatigue occur. This may seem obvious, if we don't sleep we're tired and we get depressed. We also get angry much quicker and at things that otherwise wouldn't bother us.

Spirit Sleep

Sleep is without doubt the weirdest part of our lives. It is not understood, even by the experts. I believe that the main purpose of sleep is to give our spirits a break and its equivalent of sleep. Our body repairs itself and our spirit rests.

Insufficient sleep, affects the spirit more than the body. If we can get about 8 hours uninterrupted sleep each night, our spirit and body should be perfectly recuperated each night. I can only manage about 20 minutes of uninterrupted sleep each night and so my mind, spirit and body are far from recuperated. I either give up or do the best I can, given the current circumstances.

Food to sleep by

Cherries may sound a strange item to help with sleep, yet they and grapes are a source of Melatonin, the go to sleep brain chemical.

Sugar free cherry and grape juice also work.

Another sleep helping fruit is bananas. They have potassium and magnesium, which are natural relaxants and make tryptophan.

Warm milk is a well-known sleep aid, having calcium, which relaxes us. It also has potassium and magnesium.

Toast is another strange sleep aid. It's a complex carbohydrate, which causes a sugar spike, then a crash and the production of insulin, which produces tryptophan. If we want to sleep, a crash sounds useful.

Oats, complex carbs and turkey also produce tryptophan.

Naturally, there's a but... In this case, it's eating too much or eating high protein foods which keeps us awake.

Sleep preventing foods

All the experts agree, if we want to sleep, avoid alcohol at nighttime. Obviously, don't mix alcohol and medicines, as this can be a killer, but any alcohol before bed is a problem, as our body metabolizes it quickly, causing us to wake up several times during the night. Oddly, it will make us snore or snore more and louder than usual. Other foods to avoid at bedtime are useful for production of brain chemicals we need, but they will keep us awake, as our body processes the food.

This list includes salty food, chicken, curry, dark chocolate, fatty meat and caffeine. Caffeine seems to turn up a lot. It's useful to keep us awake, but interferes with the production of our useful brain chemicals.

I can't sleep

My biggest daily issue is not being able to sleep. The worse a night I have, the less able I am to cope and the more likely I will be depressed and angry the next day. I have difficulty staying asleep, because when I'm awake I can control the pain, but not when asleep. My spirit has come up with a few methods of ensuring REM sleep, so I haven't gone completely mad. One is what I call waking dreams, where I'm watching a dream as if it was on a TV screen.

Some nights, I think I've slept for more than 20 minutes, possibly as much as a couple of hours. I'll look at the clock and see 1 minute has passed. I repeat the experience, sleeping for even longer this time, but when I look at the clock, I see the minute hand flip over from the previous minute. The night can take a long time this way. Both hips, both arms, both wrists, both hands, both knees, both ankles, my neck, stomach, chest and lower back conspire together to make sure I keep waking up. I can't lie in any position without pain. I now cover the clock so I can't see the time! If I do fall asleep, I start sweating heavily and the wet pillow, sheets and clothes I have on wake me.

I apparently get enough sleep I'm not totally crazy, but nowhere near enough to concentrate. Again, I could call a pity party and invite all my friends, all will find other engagements keep them from coming. It will also negatively charge my spirit bubble and attract negative emotions. So, I accept and celebrate **what is** and get on with my life.

So…… what am I going to do?

My "job" is to avoid all the begorphins I have mentioned over the past several pages. So something or someone wants to use begorphins to fill my spirit bubble with negative emotions … what **am I going to do** about it? The answer is to do everything I can to produce endorphins.

Service

Those who live only for themselves eventually shrivel up and figuratively lose their lives, while those who lose themselves in service to others grow and flourish—and in effect save their lives.
(Thomas S. Monson)

I have found giving service is a wonderful way to spend my time. For some reason, helping others seems to be much more fulfilling than doing things for myself.

Our brains have reward pathways, which release the feel-good chemicals into our brain when we give service to others. Giving service makes the mesolimbic pathway release oxytocin, dopamine and endorphins. Oxytocin makes us feel tranquil and serene and have a general feeling of inner peace. Dopamine and endorphins make us feel joyful and elated.

Service is the way to activate our brain's reward circuits. If our brains release dopamine, oxytocin and especially endorphins when we give service, the answer to feeling good is to give service! Doing things for ourselves doesn't have the same effect; it only works when we help others. Another one of those weird, it is what it is, aspects of the way our brain works. Service to self isn't useful to us.

The benefits of service

Studies have tried to quantify the benefits of giving. The one constant in all them is, giving service helps **us** and makes **us** feel good. Donating our time, our money, or our possessions, in a selfless way makes us feel less stressed. There is a negative link between how early we die and the amount of stress we're under. Many studies prove those who give service, live longer than those who don't.

One researcher, Jorge Moll of the D'Or Institute for Research and Education in Brazil, has shown merely by thinking about giving money to a meaningful cause, the brain releases small amounts of dopamine and endorphins. It releases a lot more when we give the money.

As well as not working when we're selfish, the brain's reward pathways don't work when we give service grudgingly. I don't know why, but only genuine, sincere, heartfelt service makes us feel better. Here's another day for me, full of service.

The radio alarm turned on the KSL morning show at 6:30am. My normal process of getting out of bed when the presenters tell me it is 6:59am doesn't always happen. Sometimes they say its 7:15am and I get out of bed as quickly as I can, which isn't very fast. I go into LLOL6's (Little Light Of my Life) bedroom, wake him, then into LLOL7's bedroom, and wake her. Next, I go down five flights of stairs to the basement, to wake LLOL5 and LLOL8. When I return to the bedroom, LLOL9 is already up and snuggling up to mom in our bed.

I dress and shower, not in that sequence, although I have had to in the past. I get dressed, get the children going, shave, undress, shower and get dressed again.

I hassle, their word not mine, the children to get dressed and have some breakfast. Many mornings, you'd think I was suggesting they eat poison, but this morning wasn't one of them. At 7:50am, I begin the task of getting the oldest four children into the car so I can take them to school. Most of you in my shoes, will know this is as easy as herding cats. I pick up the other children in the car pool and we head to school.

When I return, I finished sorting the laundry and put a load into the washer. I convince LLOL9 to get out of the bath and point her to where her clothes are, helping her button her shirt.

My wife, Ann, left for work and I put Cinderella on the TV for LLOL9. I clean the dishes off the counters, picked up random items on the landing, made Ann and LLOL9 their lunches and then got my breakfast.

This is a normal school day. If we go through this first couple of hours, I gave a lot of service this morning. I helped my five children get up and ready for school, then took them there. I did all the laundry. A normal load is only 1/7th mine, yet I did 7/7th of it. I didn't drop anything on the landing; I had not used the dishes and on and on. Yet I did it all. I refused to be acted upon by these negative ideas. I acted **as if I** want to do it all. I then found I actually did.

I'm in a lot of pain throughout the morning, yet my spirit bubble is positively charged and full of joy and happiness. This means the amount of pain I can manage is greater than when the morning began.

The right attitude

The normal drudgery of day-by-day giving doesn't necessarily activate our reward pathways, because we can easily find ourselves doing it with the wrong attitude. I can mutter and complain about having to go down five flights of stairs to wake LLOL8 and LLOL5 and then go back up those same sets of stairs to my bedroom. I could complain I need to pester the children to get ready. I could complain about being shouted at by them, as they protest I am hassling them. That I'm being a zounderkite. I can whine about having to drive them the six miles to school, even though I haven't had any breakfast, a thing I've being hassling them about for the last 30 minutes. I'm in constant pain, I haven't slept for the 5,000+ nights and last night was no better. Why can't I .....

I'll stop here. The victim-hood. bus has left and the only way forward is to look at life in a positive way regardless of the effort needed. It may take a lot of effort, but it's worth doing.

Feel good about the service I'm giving

If I want to feel good, I must feel good about giving. All I do is remind myself I am doing all this, for my wife and family, for people I love; the people I would lay my life down for; the people who are more important to me than even my own wants and needs. If they need me to be there for them, I will drop what I'm doing and do whatever I can to help them.

247

Telling myself I'm doing it all for those I love, immediately activates the reward pathways and my brain is flooded with dopamine, oxytocin and endorphins. I positively charge my spirit bubble, filling it with joy, making it possible to manage enough pain to carry on with the day.

This is how I get through every day of my life.

On the days I allow myself to be overwhelmed, my brain misses the feel-good chemicals and I feel awful. This morning, I forced myself to remember why I get up each day; why I do what I do and I felt good, almost wonderful. I'm still in pain, but I feel great nevertheless.

Many of you have similar days; especially those of you SAH parents (stay at home). As we spend time helping our family, we can remind ourselves how much we love them and that we're doing what we are, because we want to. We'll find our brain being flooded with feel good chemicals and our spirit bubble being positively charged.

Remember, we're giving service to the people we love the most. We all have a family, well most of us. Some, especially the older generation, are orphans. Some have no living children. They may not have married, or have gone through the gut-wrenching horror of having children die before them. I know our children aren't supposed to do this, but I know it happens. The world's oldest woman died in 2017, she was the last known person born in the 19th century who up till then was still alive. She had no children so we won't know whether her advanced age was genetic.

The rest of us have parents and children, nieces and nephews, aunts, uncles, cousins, in-law families, grandchildren, grandnephews and nieces. Giving service, freely and lovingly, to our families is a fantastic way to activate the reward pathways. Try it, I have and I know it works. My spirit bubble is generally full of positiveness even when I hurt. This doesn't mean that I am not attacked by negativity, it means I can beat it away.

Give to others as well

248

We can also activate the pleasure pathways by giving service to people outside of our family. The orphaned senior citizens are a perfect group to receive such service. To feel wonderful all the time, we **need** to give service to others. If you get the chance during your busy days, send me a comment on how thinking positively about what you used to consider drudgery, tiring and pointless and now consider a special responsibility, has changed your life. And all you had to do is realize the service you give to your family constantly floods our brain with feel good chemicals, reduces your stress levels, makes you feel tremendously happy and positively charges your spirit bubble.

Ann, is a teacher. One of her colleagues told of how she was getting ready for school and her first grader son said she couldn't go to school in what she was wearing, because it would embarrass him. Naturally, she didn't change and what she did was to go into his classroom after school had begun and give him a huge hug and kisses. Her spirit bubble was full of positiveness, not so sure about her son.

Taking a time-out from the children

I have learned it's no good stopping if we can't get started again. Even then, we shouldn't push past our limits, as this can be counterproductive, even when we're running at peak efficiency. When our peak is a long way from efficient, it can be dangerous, especially if driving or handling heavy machinery, or whatever else they put on the warnings for medication.

With parenting, we need to take personal time-outs to recover from looking after our children. Many days I've been out of bed for 12 to 14 hours, before I do anything for myself, except dress. I've spent all my time giving service to one or more of my children or my wife. I'm far from unique, you may have spent many days similar to this yourself and I'm sure you're grateful you can use your time this way.

One rule in place in our house, for all 130+ children is bedtime. Our goal is that 9pm is the latest our children go to their rooms and has been for nearly 40 years. We don't care if they don't go to sleep, as long as they stay in their rooms, Ann and I have about 2 hours kid-free every night. They have all complained about this relatively early watershed and we've had to explain it isn't about whether they're tired.

However we can do it, we need to take time away from our children, even if for a few hours. Date nights on a Friday is something I hear recommended a lot. You and I are different, our children are different, what we have experienced is different. How you do a time out, will be unique to you. Make sure you do, even if it's for 10 minutes walking the dog, while the children run around. Go to the shops without the children is another possibility to do something together. Ann and I value these moments whenever we can find them.

Why am I gaining weight?

What upsets me, isn't giving service to my wonderful family. It's because I don't stop, I don't get the chance to eat anything and yet, when I stand on the scales, I've put on 3 pounds. If you know who I should complain to, please email me their address. Unfortunately, it's likely to be the same person I tell my children to complain to. The Martian Ambassador to Earth.

I crashed!

At times, I find that "it" is all too much for me and no amount of positivity can overcome it. My ability to manage the pain is lower than the pain I am suffering from and heading to 10/10 across my whole body and I crash.

When this happens I have to lie down and try to sleep. I have no choice, because it doesn't matter how much, or how little pain I'm suffering, my ability to manage it is too low. The other constant when this occurs is my ability to concentrate. Or, my inability to concentrate. This is the one thing I haven't found a way to fix. When I try, I fall asleep. When my ability to manage is too low and I try, I feel dizzy and sick as well as tired.

Lying down doesn't fully help because I hurt if I lie on my back, sides or front and I can only stay asleep for a few minutes. I can't float, at least I haven't learned how to. If you know drop me an email, I might get some sleep. Lying down works because even 2 or 3 minutes of sleep helps. Over a couple of hours I may get 15 minutes of real sleep which does help me manage the pain. When I realize I've reached bottom I stop. There have been times when Ann is taking the children and dogs to the lake to swim, but, even though I want to go, I have to accept I can't. Doing more will make the pain stay high and my ability to manage it will be lower for a long time, possibly into the next day or more.

Simplify

I suffer from pain and lack of sleep, even when my children cause no stress.

Of all the humor in this book, children causing no stress, is the most ridiculous. Children and stress are inexorably connected. All of mine, whether married or not, cause me stress, as I try to balance the needs of them all. I'm not complaining, it's just is what it is.

The trick is learning to manage stress. Sounds easy. Simply manage the stress and the problems vanish. If you're living in a two-bedroom apartment and can't afford to turn the air conditioning on, or don't have any air conditioning, and your little toddler is screaming their head off, how do you manage the stress?

An easy sounding idea to reduce stress is to simplify our life. Exactly what we need when life is hard to manage. Manage the stress and the problems become easier to manage. To manage the stress we need to simplify our lives.

I checked on the Internet on simplifying our lives and was amazed at the hits. The one that intrigues me the most has 72 steps to a simpler life. Sounds like a huge amount of work to make life simpler. As well as the web sites, there are also many books on the idea of simplifying our life. If we take all the suggestions including the insane idea that we need 72 steps to simplify our life, we come down to four steps: -

1. Get organized.
2. Cut the clutter,
3. Simplify our relationships.

251

4. Slow down.

I often use the parental trick and go to the bathroom. In the 1950s they called this clocking, you didn't have to clock out, if you were using the toilet. For me, and I know for many others, this method of escape doesn't always work. The gates of Hades seem to wait for a parent to close the bathroom door, the gates open and all manner of demons escape into your house.

At other times, the children have no concept of privacy. If we invade their private space when they are enthroned, they scream and shout for us to leave. If we're enthroned, the King or Queen is available and can't escape. As a child wants and needs attention, they rightly work out we cannot escape, or give someone else our attention. With my children, this generally stops when they reach about eight and believe it too gross to do anymore. I can't recall a time when there wasn't someone younger than eight in my family.

Ann and I try to take time away from the children whenever we can. She has a 30-minute lunch break. I meet her at school and we have lunch together. When our parents were close by, we'd drop the children off with them for a while. We are weird; we're the grandparents of nine and have five angels in training still at home. Our married children often want to use us as the drop off station.

We did this with them. And now they want some kid-free time.

It's essential our spirit bubbles are positively charged when dealing with children. We need to be happy and joyful so they can be. Otherwise, they become victims of "don't let mum brush your hair when she is upset!" syndrome.

Neurotransmitter creation

I can't take a time-out each time I feel down because I'd be in permanent time-out, so a different type of stress management is necessary. I do all I can to keep the endorphins flowing along with the dopamine and the serotonin.

I tend to go up to about 30% during the day. That's approximately 30% of my best, prior to the car wreck in 2002. I keep my spirit in the captain's chair and do the best I can to feel happy and be joyful.

This sounds like a whine, even to me. We have a sign over our back door, which says, "Thou shalt not whine", so let's try that again. Mornings are problematical, regardless of when I get out of bed, but at least I have a reason to do so. In fact, several reasons. In 2017, my reasons are aged 17, 15, 14, 13 and 7, or as I have titled them LLOL5 through 9. (**Little Light Of my Life**)

Having children in my life gives me a purpose, a reason to carry on with life. I can't speculate on whether I'd get up without them because, as I say to my teenage son when he starts the "what if" questioning. I answer with a question of my own. "What if a number 205 bus fell from the sky onto your head?" He generally finds my question unhelpful and what he calls rude.

Hang on a second

You may have noticed I haven't answered the questions of how to manage stress or how to simplify my life. That's because I can't give you a good answer to them. I take each day at a time and do whatever I can to lower the stress levels and simplify my life and positively charging my spirit bubble. I am aware of my need to do so and this seems to work for me. Not always, but enough I'm not raving mad. I checked with my married niece and she agrees I'm simply mad.

Being a Parent

Since you get more joy out of giving joy to others, you should put a good deal of thought into the happiness that you're able to give. (Eleanor Roosevelt)

As family is my reason for continuing, for staying the course let me share some more stories about my children. Being distracted, helps to lower my pain and what better distraction is there than children?

Not all agree.

Jaelyn had come to live with us when she was two days old, the eighth child of her 31-year-old mother. Number 7 had died in somewhat strange circumstances and all the others had been removed. Yet, here she was with number eight being taken away. Mother and child both tested positive for cocaine, so Jaelyn automatically came into care and came to live with us.

Mother wasn't bothered or interested in what happened to her daughter. "Oh well, let me know" was her response to being told she was losing her baby. When asked about setting up visits, as mandated by the courts, she responded, "It doesn't matter, just call me." She'd lost seven children and this one was of no more interest to her. It was just an inconvenience.

Pregnancy was an unpleasant bi-product of her life style. She was a drug user, who cared nothing about the children who were the result of "buying" the drugs. She felt no responsibility and didn't even consider trying to ensure no more children were conceived.

A selfish person's spirit bubble

Her spirit bubble could be viewed as confusing to anyone else. A selfish person's bubble seems to have another bubble inside of it. A tiny self-contained bubble with feel-good emotions from which they try to feed constantly. The rest of their bubble is filled with negativity.

The drugs directly feed the self-contained bubble and can help them feel positive for a short while. When the drugs wear off, the whole bubble turns black and is "mega-negative" Jaelyn had been with us for three months and we'd helped her through her addiction withdrawals and a fight with RSV, a lung disease with a high mortality rate. We now had a heartbreaking choice.

Do you want another?

One month after we'd adopted Emily, we received a phone call from the hospital where she'd been born. The social worker on duty knew us and left a confusing message.

She said, "she was the case worker on the err, um, err, case I'm working on." She apparently didn't want to tell us who. She waffled on for some minutes, before telling us she wanted to know if we were interested in taking a sibling of a baby, and she said Emily's birth name. We had to assume she meant either, Emily's biological mum had had another baby, or they needed to move one of her three older biological siblings. She'd called at 4:45pm, and then went home.

We called back the next day and she told us Emily's mother had walked into the hospital with a baby girl saying she "didn't want her." Many US states have an abandonment law allowing a mother to go to a police station, a fire station, a hospital or a government office and hand over a newborn baby. The only question asked is the mother's name. The laws are there to try to stop the too common occurrence of babies being found in dumpsters.

The worker asked us if we wanted the baby. We couldn't take her then, as she was critically ill. She wanted us to know, so we could contact the CPS office and get the wheels moving, if we wanted to, err um, ok?

The next day, we went to the CPS office to get more details on the baby. Our social worker laughingly warned us not to go across the road to the hospital. Naturally, we ignored her. We were ushered into a room where a small pediatric intensive care crib was in the corner. Through the window, we could see the nursery with all the brightly

255

colored cribs holding the recently born babies. This room was cold and antiseptic with bright lights and sinks, benches and extra equipment

We put on one of those wonderful backless things and the nurse handed the baby to Ann. She held her for some minutes then let me. She was tiny and had a name tag of "baby girl" on her ankle. Those first few hugs were enough to convince us. We had to make her our own. Our spirit bubbles had been filled with love from the brief time we had been blessed to hold her. She still fills my spirit bubble.

We'll take her

We returned to the CPS office and told the social worker what she already knew. In the few hours we'd been gone, she'd begun the process of getting a variance on our fostering license. Taking her meant we'd have too many children in our home. With earlier babies, we'd taken the baby first and then a variance. This time we did it the right way around. It took nearly a week to get approval.

In an odd set of circumstances, she wasn't delivered to our home. I drove to a strip mall, twenty miles from home and met the social worker there. She handed the baby over to me at a toy store.

Now, we had our two adopted children, two-year-old Matthew, one-year-old Emily and now her newborn baby sister. We also had six-year-old Bagley and of course, three-month-old Jaelyn. Our foster care license allowed us to have six children, so we were all right there. We were allowed two babies, less than eighteen months old and we now had three, making us one baby too many. The variance resolved the difficulty for us for a while.

What a choice we had to make!

It was obvious Jaelyn wasn't heading home and needed a long-term permanent placement. We hope a family member can take the child. In Jaelyn's case, her mother proved the maxim of the apple doesn't fall far from the tree. Her father could have been anyone of men, so that was a dead end.

We had the right to adopt her, if we wanted to. Otherwise, we had to sign a form specifically saying we didn't. She was nearly three months old and already recognized everybody. She could almost roll over and chattered non-stop, in a deep, throaty, sexy voice. We had to decide whether we could cope with four children so close in age, for the next twenty or more years. This was the subject of much discussion and prayer. Eventually we came to the distressing decision we couldn't deal with their complicated issues.

We had to choose between Jaelyn and Lucy. As we already had her sister, we chose Lucy and later adopted her. We signed the relinquishment forms and began looking for someone to take Jaelyn. Normally CPS did this, but Ann was president of the Foster Parent's Association and we knew most of the foster parents. Jaelyn left us 10 weeks later; she left to live with a wonderful family.

We believe this was Heavenly Father's plan all along and we were only her temporary home. As with many other children, we'd helped her through many significant problems her new family may not have been able to manage. Our spirit bubbles were filled with sad and happy thoughts at the same time. In the end, the happy thoughts won out.

Detour

We took a detour on our trip down the mountain and across the desert. What at first seemed to be the wrong road, turned out to be a diversion to pick up someone who needed our help. A child we would take into our family and make our own. We'd do all we could to fix her, so they could safely continue on the road without us.

We found joy in pain, knowing Jaelyn had found a forever family. We were happy for her. We also found joy in adding another daughter, Lucy, to our growing family. We made our spirit bubble positively charged by concentrating on the positives of what happened.

Ann and I picked up 130+ hitchhikers and for a while, ranging from 1 day to forever, welcomed them into our home and family. Not a bad set of detours, or a bad set of decisions either, even with the responsibilities they have brought. If I could do it all again, I believe I'd make the same choices and the same detours.

Mad?

257

Many people have told us we're totally mad. Maybe we are. I'm in a lot of pain and can no longer work. Yet we keep on fostering.

Ann broke her neck in the March 2002 accident and was in a metal halo for several months. This device has six metal rods screwed into the skull to hold the halo in place. A breastplate and back plate make sure your neck and the halo can't move. When you lie down, your head is suspended six inches from the bed or pillow and Ann tells me it's horrific. You lie on your back whether you want to or not. She now had a halo and this means she must be an angel, although instead of just hanging a few inches above her head, it was screwed into her skull. Even though she was still wearing this Inquisition style device, we were fostering again. It was 9 months before I could use my left arm and yet we were at it again.

We were giving a home, love and care to children who, through no fault of their own, were living lives of hell. We were finding joy in pain, mad or not. I know those who think we're mad could not fill their spirit bubbles with positiveness and joy by taking these children, but I can and I have.

We're praying for you

After the March 2002 accident, we found help through this traumatic time, when strangers came up and told us they were praying for us. The fact people were thinking about us made us feel better. This sort of faith works whether you believe in God or not. Positive vibes, or whatever you want to call them, seem to help. I know they did for us. By August, Amy was back at school and in the color guard. Ann had the halo removed in June and Andrew was back to normal by September. They'd gone through $2,000,000 of medical treatment and had recovered within 6 months. I broke my arm and years later, I've yet to recover, but it is what it is.

Our foster children have also benefited from prayer and the positive vibes in our home, from us having positively charged spirit bubbles. Within two or three days, a child with sunken eyes, who won't even look at you, changes into a bright-eyed fun loving little person. The child, who can't believe we're feeding her again, when we had fed her this morning and at lunchtime, learns they get fed more than once every few days.

They stapled who to what??

We had a harder job with 3-year-old Tonia and her fear of closed doors. She came to us when police found her and her 18-month-old brother wandering naked around the street. They couldn't find their parents, so they called CPS.

The first night with us, Tonia woke up at 2am and started screaming incoherently. This happened for several nights; before I worked out she wanted the door open. The fact the door was open, made the problem hard to resolve.

We eventually found out what scared her so much. Her parents stapled her to the bedroom door, when they wanted to go out and party. She'd stay fastened to the door until they came home again and pulled the staples out. I find it hard to believe her parents could do something as appalling, yet they did.

Her father, who we'll call Richard, was arrested not long after he lost his children, while target practicing with his rifle in a public park. He had placed the target near a path and a teenager passed in front of it, so Richard shot him, twice. His reasoning? The kid crossed in front of the target so Richard had no choice but to shoot him. The police and courts decided to make sure Richard couldn't own a gun again.

It didn't take too long to calm Tonia down and even allow the bedroom door to be closed. She trusted us, she believed what we were saying and I no longer had to get up at 2am to convince her, an open door was really open. I poked through the door, walked in and out of it, shut the door and reopened it. None of these initially worked and she just kept on screaming that she wanted the door open.

I admit being forced out of bed, because a child is screaming, was having a serious effect on my spirit bubble and filling it with irritation and some anger. Finding and solving the problem positively filled both mine and Tonia's.

A day in Ann's life

259

Ann and I fostered both sides of the accident in 2002 with as many foster children since as we had before. We began fostering in 1991 in England. We moved to Texas in 1997 and in 2000, were fostering in Dallas. We moved to Utah in 2005 and started fostering again the next year. Once we started taking foster children, our lives became different from most people our age. Initially, we were taking foster children a few years younger than our own children. Now we were in Texas, our children were 9 years older and our foster children were still younger than our children had been 9 years previously. In Utah, the same has been true. My youngest adopted child is 5 years younger than my oldest grandchild is.

You can expect a measure of chaos in our house most of the time. It goes with the territory of children with ruined lives, too often ruined before they were even born. Here is Ann's write up for an average day in our house.

It's 6.29 am and I drag myself out of bed and down three flights of stairs to the basement to start the morning routine. Four-year-old Rosita is awake and happy to see me, but nine-year-old Anastasia isn't. She gripes, whines, and wishes the bus wouldn't come at 7.30am. I don't have time to discuss anything with her, upstairs two-year-old John is screaming at the top of his lungs because six-year-old Lisa has told him to get out of her room.

In the next room, Emma's bed is wet and she's smelly. At seven, she's embarrassed she still pees the bed, so she tries to hide the dirty pull-up and Dave goes on a search for it. I fill the bathtub and point Emma in the right direction. Dave pulls the soaking bed covers towards the laundry room and I go into Michael's room tentatively.

Michael is an unknown quantity in the morning – sweet and co-operative, or a wild animal. You don't know what you'll find on the top bunk. I do know the bedroom he shares with John will be trashed. After we put him to bed he'll have retrieved his secret stash of tortilla chips, ate and scrunched them. Scattered them like snowflakes from the top bunk, tipped up all the toy boxes and pulled

260

the books from the bookshelf. John enjoys this – he can find a new toy every morning to drag into the living room or leave on the stairs.

I ask Dave to go find Michael's medicine and use every persuasive tone I can manage to persuade the eight-year-old to get out of bed. When all else fails, I go to my room to see if the girls have appeared yet, leaving Dave to do what he can to perform a miracle to get Michael to the bus on time.

As I try to fix hair for the three older girls, Rosita and John open and close all the drawers in my room and slam doors at each other. Eventually they're screaming again and I can barely hear little Nina who has woken in her bassinet and wants me to know when you're merely ten weeks old, you like it if someone feeds you when you wake. Eventually we make it down to the kitchen. It's 7.03.

We pull out ten boxes of cereal because everyone wants something different. Rosita and John will eat four bowls each, spilling at least two. The others are frantically trying to find a matching pair of socks. They remember they left their shoes by the trampoline last night and the sprinklers have recently soaked them. We now have a mad search for alternative footwear.

I'm feeding the baby, sweet little thing, when we notice the atmosphere smells suspicious. Rosita, John and Nina all need diaper changes – the first three diapers of the morning are taken to the trash can which is already overflowing and its five days till the men come to empty it.

Michael is calming down a bit now and wants to play with John and the dog. They start running around the living room. Anastasia is ready when the neighborhood kids knock on the door, but Michael is still missing his shoes, his backpack and his jacket. He yells no one is helping him, and then asks John if he wants to go to school with him. John does, but he's only two and still in pajamas. When I say he can't go, the screaming starts again and Rosita joins in because she doesn't want to be left out. We push Anastasia and Michael out the door with kisses, while trying to stop the dog, John and Rosita from following them.

We breathe a sigh of relief for a moment. It's short lived. Lisa and Emma choose this moment to produce all the homework they insisted they didn't have yesterday and announce they need something for bring and share. While I try to tidy the kitchen, grateful for a dog to lick the milk off the floor, Dave goes at the homework and tries to explain to the toddlers we don't want to watch Clifford the Big Red Dog. John takes this reasonably and spends the next thirty minutes lining up toy cars on the kitchen table so Rosita can mess them up later and bring on another tantrum. Nina is fed now, but wants to go back to sleep and I haven't had a chance to bathe her yet.

I try to distract Rosita from Clifford by suggesting she go take a bath, she likes the idea and so does John, and so we head upstairs. We must go to the DCFS office today to visit with their mother. It's a sixty-mile round trip and we need to be there by 10.00am. We're on a roll today and it's only 8.07.

"I love you Mom" Emma calls to me as I struggle to wash Rosita's hair. She and Lisa head for the school bus, so as soon as they're gone, Dave comes upstairs to help dress the three remaining kids.

Three kids are no big deal, we can do it in a flash, but then John gets into Emma's play make up and needs cleaning and clean clothes again. Rosita poops again the minute she's in a clean pull up.

There are four baskets of laundry this morning, plus Emma's bed covers. Dave makes a start, while I hit the shower, but I find it difficult to relax when I know the door will burst open at any minute, or the third world war will break out in the kitchen.

I rush to dress and blow-dry my hair in record time, while trying to keep little hands from raiding my make-up drawer. Niña was asleep in her crib, but Rosita enjoys poking her and soon she's crying. I console her and lay her back down, Rosita has my hairbrush now and it's stuck in her hair.

It's 8.29. Dave and I've been awake for two hours, we have changed seven diapers, fixed five lots of hair, bathed three kids, fed seven, cleaned a kitchen, put in laundry, helped with homework, changed bed sheets, got four to school, swept the floor, policed at least five skirmishes and given medication to two children.

Just a snapshot

This is one tiny snapshot of our lives. It isn't an exaggeration, if anything we have underestimated the amount of work Ann and I do in our home each morning. Some mornings aren't as stressful.

Occasionally, the children all get up, get dressed, come downstairs and get breakfast, finish their homework and leave for the school bus without any problems. They sit and cuddle with Ann as she feeds the baby and they are all kind and considerate.

With five children, this may seem to be a miracle, but it happens regularly. As do the stressful days.

Why I get out of bed

This is why I get out of bed in the morning. I don't fall asleep until 5am and getting up at 6:30am may seem silly, but I have purpose to my day. I'm not simply a person with over 50 broken bones, all of which still hurt. I'm someone who must get up and put on the role of dad for the rest of the day.

Our experience, with children of all ages, has taught us when we're a parent; we realize that even though we're running as fast as we can, we can't seem to get anywhere.

We find ourselves sitting in a school hall, listening to awful music being played by children, some of whom are smaller than their musical instruments.

We willingly watch badly acted plays and cheer wildly at the end and not because it's over. We freeze to death watching Football games in the middle of winter.

Fighting Pain Finding Joy

Our child is playing on the school team, or is in the band, the color guard, the cheer-leading group or is selling drinks at the concession stand. We ignore the fact that few, if any, of the players on either team can catch the ball, even if it had a homing device and Velcro. We may wonder how we finished off there. When we think about it, we realize we want to be there.

They're our children, our pride and joy and we're there to support them. It has made no difference to Ann or to me we weren't these children's biological parents. We are giving service to people who we love and are filling both our and their spirit bubbles with joy.

We willingly accept the role of taxi driver, traveling in ever decreasing circles; taking one child to the doctors, another to the dentist, one to gymnastics, another to baseball and another to soccer, all at the same time. What feels like a fleeting time later, we do it all in reverse, to pick them up again. Many times, having fed them, we put them all to bed. I once drove 165 miles between 8am and 4pm, being no more than 8 miles from home. This is in addition to being chief cook, bottle washer, nurse, etc. etc. Once we have been a parent for a while, we realize there are many et ceteras. We have conversations with two-year old's, never sure of the topic. We also have conversations with our teenagers and are even more confused about the topic.

Even though in our case, most of our children didn't begin life as ours, they've come into our lives hoping we'd pretend they had, that we'd "act as if" they had. They have come into the world in the same way every other baby has. For some reason, their biological parents can't or won't accept the responsibility of caring properly for them and the state steps in. Some have come to live with us, bringing with them their emotional, mental and spiritual pain and, at times, physical pain. Their spiritual bubbles are full of negativity. Our job has been to teach them to fill their bubbles with positivity.

We've fulfilled the role of parents for as long as we need to do for all of our children, forever for 9 of them. We adopted 6 of our children from foster care. If this makes me stupid, I admit it, not only am I

264

empty headed, as proved by the nose surgeries. If it is stupid then it's the most wonderful stupid I can find. You can get me my sign and I will proudly display it.

Stupid?

Talking of people who deserve the "here's your sign" for stupid statements. I'm amazed how many there are.

Abuse is no respecter of race, gender or social status and we often have a veritable United Nations in our house.

Our adopted children are a mix of Asian, African American, Caucasian and Latino. Many times, we've had three babies, one black, one white and one brown. People have asked us if they're triplets, despite the fact they don't look the same, are different colors and most often different ages. One foster mother we know, when asked this question, agreed they were indeed triplets and told the person asking, this is what happens when you fool around. Another claimed she'd checked them out of the library. My favorite response has been to ask how they guessed.

A new child preparation program

For some time, a tongue in cheek instruction sheet preparing people to become parents has been circulating on the Internet It gets so many search hits, it's difficult, if not impossible, to find the original author. I've changed the list to include the knowledge Ann and I have garnered in 40+ years of being parents to our 130+ children. I include it because it's funny. When I need to laugh, this is one of the places I go. It's helped me with fighting pain finding joy, as it fills my spirit bubble with joy and happiness. Enjoy.

* Children are an expensive commodity. Go to the grocery store and arrange to have your salary paid directly to their head office. This will make it easier, when you find little money left, once you've bought food. Baby milk costs at least $25 a can. Much more, for the special milk. You'll need at least 9 or 10 cans a month. Diapers cost

40c to 70c each diaper and you'll need six or more each day, per child.

* As well as costing a lot of money, children are time expensive. You'll find little time left over to spend on your favorite pastimes. If you enjoy keeping up with current events, you'll need to spend all the time between now and the birth of your baby, either reading newspapers, or logging on to your favorite web news site.

* You need to do this step before the baby is born. Find a couple who already are parents and berate them about their...
- *Methods of discipline.*
- *Lack of patience.*
- *Appallingly low tolerance levels.*
- *Allowing their children to run wild.*
- *Suggest ways in which they might improve their child's breastfeeding, sleep habits, toilet training, table manners, and overall behavior. Enjoy it, because it will be the last time in your life, you'll have all the answers.*

* Sleep is necessary to ensure we can think clearly and being a new parent needs a clear mind. To get a good idea how your nights will be, when you bring home your pride and joy, do the following.
- *As soon as you get home from work, begin walking around the living room, carrying a wet bag weighing approximately 8-12 pounds. Do this from 5pm to 10pm with a radio tuned to static or some other obnoxious sound. At the same time, eat cold food with one hand.*
- *At 10PM, gently lay the bag down; set the alarm for midnight, and go to sleep.*
- *When the alarm sounds, get up, lift the bag up, walk around the living room until 1AM. Gently lay the bag back down.*
- *Set the alarm for 3AM and go back to bed. Because you've been woken up, you'll find you can't get back to sleep. So, get up at 2AM, make a drink and watch a cartoon.*

- *Go to bed at 2:45AM.*
- *Get up at 3AM when the alarm goes off. Sing songs quietly in the dark until 4AM.*
- *At 6am, get up, make breakfast, get ready and go to work. You'll need to work hard and be productive.*

Repeat these steps each night for 3-5 years (1 year for each child you later have.) Don't forget to look cheerful and together, always.

* *Children are messy. They must learn how to be tidy. To get an idea of how it feels to have children, follow these steps.*

- *Smear peanut butter onto the sofa and onto the curtains.*
- *Hide a piece of raw chicken behind the TV and leave it there all summer.*
- *Stick your fingers in the flowerbed, and rub them on the clean walls.*
- *Take your favorite book, photo album, etc. Pull pages out, tearing pages or drawing all over them.*
- *Spill milk on your new pillows and cover the stains with crayons.*
- *Take all your small ornaments and destroy them.*

* *Dressing small children isn't as easy as it seems. To learn how, perform the following steps until you're an expert.*

- *Buy an octopus and a small bag made from loose mesh. Put the octopus into the bag so no arms hang out.*
- *To get a feeling for how easy it can be to change a child, especially a tired, cranky and hungry one, select two legs and tie a large dishtowel around the bottom of the legs. The legs should be from opposite sides of the octopus.*
- *If you've been married for some time, before you have your first child, you'll probably have a nice car. Sell it. You may want to buy a car previously owned by a family.*

* *One of the time-tested ways of proving your parenting credentials is to take one or more little children to the grocery store. If you don't*

have a child, find the closest thing you can to a pre-school child. A full-grown goat is an excellent choice. If you intend to have more than one child, take more than one goat. Buy your week's groceries without letting the goats out of your sight. Pay for everything the goat eats or destroys. Until you can easily do this, don't even contemplate having children.

* *Even though a baby has four basic skills, eating, sleeping, crying and voiding (pooping and peeing), feeding a baby is so difficult it should be an Olympic event. The following steps will train you for feeding a nine-month-old baby.*

- *Hollow out a melon, make a small hole in the side and suspend it from the ceiling using string or rope.*
- *Swing it from side to side.*
- *Get a bowl of soggy cereal and try to spoon the cereal into the swaying melon by pretending to be an airplane.*
- *Continue until half the cereal is gone. Tip half into your lap and throw the rest up in the air.*

* **Being** *a parent often seems to be contradictory. We look forward to the day they begin talking, then wish they'd be quiet. To understand how this works, make a recording of someone you find irritating saying 'mommy' or "daddy" repeatedly. There should be no more than a four-second delay between each 'mommy' or "daddy". Every so often, increase the volume to 100%. Play the recording in your car, everywhere you go for the next four years. You're now ready to take a trip with a toddler. After eighteen months, add the word 'why' every 30 seconds.*

* *Being able to have an intelligent conversation with another adult becomes increasingly difficult, as your child gets older. This is especially true when trying to use the telephone. To understand how this one works, start talking to an adult of your choice. Have someone continually tug on your skirt hem, shirtsleeve, or elbow while playing the 'mommy' recording. You're now ready to have a conversation with an adult, with a child in the room.*

I hope you enjoyed reading how to be a parent. If you already have children, you know I'm right. Despite it all, I insist it is all worth it.

Foster children

When the child is a foster child, who has come from a life you may find incomprehensible; life can be even harder and weirder. Most of our children have come to live with us as babies, 62 as newborns. We've been through the program many times. For two years, we had a newborn baby constantly. Not the same one, obviously. We'd get a baby, help them through the withdrawals and teach them how to sleep the night. If it took us more than two weeks to have them sleep the night, we were doing something wrong. By between 6 and 12 weeks, DCFS would have found a family member to take them and from 2 to 6 weeks later, they'd leave us. In the meantime, we'd have taken another newborn into our house. Our spirit bubbles were constantly being filled with the joy of having a newborn baby.

Children have helped me with fighting pain finding joy and positively charging my spirit bubble with that joy. I can forget my own physical, emotional, spiritual and emotional pain by concentrating on fixing theirs.

You may have a completely different method of filling your spirit bubble. You may believe my method would fill yours with massive amounts of negativity. That is okay. What works for me, works for me. Don't simply ignore my idea and not bother to find what works for you.

It may take some time, but whatever helps you fight pain and find joy and fills your bubble with positive emotions, with joy do it. Whatever makes it possible for you to fill other people's bubbles with joy, do it. Begorphins only exist in a negative state, there are no positive begorphins. If there are begorphins around us, our spirit bubbles will be negatively charged.

Be warned. Substance abuse **does not work**. Drugs and drug abuse have brought 130+ children to our family and why there are

480,000 children in the foster care system in the United States alone. Substance abuse ruins the lives of everyone involved. Parents and children included.

Selfishness doesn't work either. What works is giving service in as many ways as we can. Almost any begorphin can be overcome by giving service.

A Second Is All It Takes

Happiness can be hard to find, but it is worth the search.
(David Gray)

A couple of the car accidents I've had, have occurred because of split second decisions. In England, I was driving home one night and needed to make a turn onto a different road. A car decided not to bother waiting for me to complete the maneuver, which involved crossing in front of his car. He told me his foot slipped and that was why his car shot straight into the side of my car. Had his foot decided to slip a few seconds later, I'd have been gone, or a few seconds earlier, his car would have shot out in front of me and I'd have swerved to avoid him. Slipping when it did, ensured an accident. I had a tough time convincing the other driver he was at fault. Fortunately, his insurance company didn't

I had an accident in 2007, as I was traveling northbound on I-15 near Ogden, Utah. The vehicles in front of me stopped when a construction truck pulled onto the central median area.

The transportation department in Utah seems to have spent the past 40 years doing road works on I-15 in Utah. This predilection for doing road works is, of course, the reason transportation departments exist throughout the world. It has been estimated the sun will last for another 2.5 billion years, meaning our local highway departments will be completing the road works in the dark.

The moron in charge

I was once stuck in a traffic jam caused by road works. The traffic lights had been set in such a way cars couldn't get through the junction before the light changed back to red. Once I eventually got through and to work, I called the local city's transportation department and asked to speak to the moron in charge of the road works. They put me straight through to someone. I was impressed no one thought it odd

I asked for the chief moron. At least someone came and reset the traffic lights so there was not gridlock each morning and afternoon.

Don't follow the trucks

These road works on I-15, this morning were making the road wider and several trucks, made up of three trailers, were taking part in the construction. They were too long to pull straight into the center and had to stop with the first two trailers off the road and the third in the carriageway. The other carriageway was closed and there were only two lanes open, one southbound and the one I was in, heading northbound.

I saw a sign warning not to follow construction vehicles. I was confused, but looking ahead, I realized what was meant. Four cars ahead, a truck had pulled the first two trailers off and had stopped, with the third trailer in the carriageway. The cars in front of me stopped. I was traveling at 55mph and was standing up to push on the brakes, trying to bring my 1-ton Suburban to a stop. I stopped inches from the car in front of me. The car behind me didn't stop and hit my car with enough force, despite the fact I had the brakes full on, to push me forward into the vehicle in front. I was whiplashed into the steering wheel, and then pushed back into the seat, forcing me to sit back down, then forward and back at least once more.

I walked around to the back to see what had happened and to chew out the idiot who had hit me. Behind me was a red saloon, completely squashed from front bumper to the driver and passenger seats. The air bags had deployed and the driver was next to the car. As I looked over at the passenger seat, a screaming teenage girl got out the car. She didn't seem to realize, or remember, there were cars heading southbound at 55mph or greater in the lane next to us. She was about to step into the path of a car when I shouted and jumped at her, pulling her back. I looked at the back of my car and was surprised there seemed to be no damage to it.

The point of this story is the choices made in it. Unbelievably, the woman driving the car that hit mine, told me the first sign she had I was stopping, was when my brake lights came on. As this is their purpose, it made no sense that she chose to continue at 55 mph, instead of choosing to hit the brakes. She had a split second to decide and she made the wrong one. I also had a split-second decision to make, regarding the young woman in the passenger seat of the car. Had I made the wrong decision, she'd have been a hood ornament on one of the cars heading the other way and undoubtedly would have died.

I have found that having the brakes full on, won't necessarily stop the opposing forces from pushing against us. Hopefully our plan of happiness has instructions on how to deal with this sort of problem. If not, we can find ourselves pushed off a cliff.

Pain under control

My spirit was in the captain's chair and overriding all the pain messages my neck and lower back were sending into the control center. This is because I had something much more important to manage, my 6-year-old son Matthew. For an hour, my spirit had complete control of the whole pain management systems of my body. As soon as we got home, it relaxed and I realized how much I was hurting and I went to the emergency room. The accident caused me a lot of pain, which I'm still suffering from.

I suffered through months of torture at the hands of pain clinic staff, to finish off with pain in my neck and lower back, which is where I was before they did anything. You can't imagine, unless you have been through it, how hard it is lying on a bed in a room full to overflowing with medical students, while having a stellate ganglion block with no anesthetic.

The doctor told me not to move, while he pushed a 6-inch needle into my neck from the front aiming for a nerve bundle at the back, using the images from a real-time x-ray machine, which took up ¾ of the room. He warned me not to move, or I may be paralyzed and not to talk, because he might hit my vocal chords and I'd probably not talk again. Swallowing and breathing were also not recommended. The block causes a Horner's syndrome, numbing me from shoulder to fingertips and upwards towards my head. The idea is to turn off all the pain receptors and when the numbness wears off, the pain has gone.

None worked. Once the numbness and pins and needles wore off and I had the use of the left side of my face, the pain in my upper arm returned, often with a vengeance. The ones done in my lower back, given to try to stop the pain in my IS joint, also failed. These differed only in the fact the warnings didn't include not swallowing.

Eventually, after a block didn't even cause a Horner's syndrome, one of the doctors told me, and I quote, "we haven't done s**t for you, have we?" and he suggested I stop going. To make me feel even better, when I reached a settlement with the insurance company of the woman who was driving the other car, Medicare insisted I paid most of the settlement to them, for the treatment. Once all the other medical organizations and my lawyers took their 40% cut, I effectively got $0 as my share. Nothing about it gave me any joy. My life with RSD!

This doesn't mean I should give up, it just means that, out of a horrible situation, all we may get is unpleasantness and pain. It gives me, what we might call the parameters I now deal with and within to meet the needs of my personal plan of happiness.

I keep looking for new and innovative ways to fight the pain, find joy and positively charge my spirit bubble. At the same time I have to ignore the negativeness that comes, when things don't improve.

Autopilot

Joy is increased by giving it to others (Robert McCheyne)

With most of the things we do each day like breathing, walking, knowing where we are in space etc., the everyday activities, we learn how to do everything so well, we allow ourselves to run on autopilot. There is no one in the captain's chair and everything is running using the programming we've previously created. The fancy term for this is autonomic.

Sometimes, we aren't prepared for what happens, especially when it comes to pain. As we've grown older, we've also become wiser. We know not to touch hot things; although we may manage to accidentally. We may have some pre-programmed processes to limit the pain. Put burned hand under cold tap, put lavender on the burn, etc. If it's bad enough we may decide to go to the hospital. When I set fire to my face, I did all I could and then went to the nearest emergency room to get treatment from an expert.

I can't breathe

There are times when we've no routines ready to run, because we've not previously experienced what's happening. At 16, I woke up with a horrendous pain in my chest. I realized I couldn't breathe without intense pain. I had pleurisy, and over the next several days, was in pain with every breath or drugged, so I felt nothing at all. Around the lungs, preventing them from rubbing against our ribs is the pleural lining. When the lining dries out, we have pleurisy and our lungs rub against the ribs, causing the agony.

My spirit was now fully awake and busy. Unfortunately, it had a conundrum to deal with. The system in charge of pain management was receiving messages from the ribs on the lower left quadrant concerning torture every time I breathed. The override button was pushed on the breathing console saying, "hold your breath!"

Not surprisingly, alarm bells sounded from all stations, as they all need fresh oxygen and for the carbon dioxide to be expelled. Each was sending a loud request for intervention. As soon as an override button was pressed, the system reset and re-sounded the alarm for some other part of my body.

Our muscles need a lot of oxygen to work. Our brain needs even more. But it hurt to breathe! I was stuck in an impossible quandary, trying to decide whether I should breathe in or suffer the pain doing so would cause.

Computer chaos

I've been in a computer control room when this sort of chaos occurred. In the early 1970s, I worked for Coutts Bank, the most prestigious bank in London and probably the world. All the bank's branches were connected to the computer department. Each branch had a set of lights and switches, with which we could check its network status. I was working with a junior operator, who had left the master computer console open. I'll not go into the history and management of early Univac computers. Suffice to say, this was potentially catastrophic for the network. I happened to be standing near the network panel and noticed the lights were slowing down across the board.

I moved out, so I could see the console and saw the console light was flashing. I shouted to Daniel, who was sitting at the console, to release the console lock. This is a computer speak for "push the flashing button."

Everything slowed for a moment, as I saw him reach over to the main power button. The console with the flashing light was on the left. The power button was on the bottom right of the large unit on the right. We didn't press it unless we were doing preventative maintenance and needed to reset the whole computer system. If the network was live, the only phrase that fits is "all hell breaks loose". Every alarm sounded and as each branch had an alarm connected to the line, the noise was mind bending.

I quickly ran to the console and, pushing Daniel aside, began turning the system back on. The alarms I left sounding. My boss came running in to see what had happened. I told him Daniel had turned the computer off. Daniel tried to blame me, saying I'd told him to do it. I argued I'd told him to clear the console.

My boss told some other computer operators to shut the alarms off and asked me how long before the network was back up. I told him 15 minutes and continued running the necessary programs. He called security and had Daniel escorted off the premises. This sort of stupidity was a fireable offense and my boss had no problem with it.

Chaos in the control room of my brain

This chaos is what was happening in the control room of my brain. I didn't dare breathe, because it hurt too much. I **had** to breathe though, I needed the oxygen. Even trying to breathe shallowly wasn't working, even that hurt. Eventually, I managed to crawl into my parents' bedroom and whimper for help. One called a doctor, who came out, diagnosed pleurisy, and gave me a shot for the pain.

Heart Attack?

This sort of decision-making is the way pain management has become for me all the time now. For example, when an alarm bell goes off in the chest area. My app knows to check the symptoms for a heart attack: -

- *chest pain,*
- *shoulder pain.*
- *pain in the left arm,*
- *sweating;*
- *restricted feeling, as if someone had tied a rope around your chest and back,*
- *fatigue,*
- *shortness of breath,*
- *flu like symptoms,*
- *dizziness,*

- *anxiety,*
- *insomnia.*

Our app reports to the spirit whether the symptoms match or not. If the symptoms match but go away, we may decide it isn't a heart attack and we keep trying to work out what's causing the pain. If we've been running, we may have a stitch and should stop running and walk until the pain subsides. It could be spicy food and we do whatever we do about that. And so on. If there are no other possibilities, we should call for an ambulance. Waiting for the symptoms to go away can have deadly results. If it is a heart attack, the result could well be death.

Is Ann having a heart attack or not?

On the day after Christmas 2016, Boxing Day, my wife experienced many symptoms listed for a heart attack and I took her to the doctors on December 27. He told her it was a heart attack, did an EKG and took a blood sample to do an enzyme test to make sure it was.

Over the next few weeks, into the middle of February, she had nuclear medicine, stress test and whatever else the doctors thought might help. The x-rays seemed to show a blocked artery in the heart and she was scheduled for an angiogram and putting in a stent to fix the blockage. The angiogram showed there was nothing wrong with her heart. The doctor told us to go away and, oh, here's a huge bill.

She suffered through endoscopies at both ends of her alimentary canal and to cut a long and expensive story short, the cure was some ant-acid medication available over-the-counter for a few dollars. All that worry and money because the symptoms matched something truly horrible.

I have those symptoms all the time

For me, my left arm hurts all the time; my chest hurts all the time, often a huge amount. In fact, the only symptom I don't have all the time is shortness of breath. I've needed to rewrite the "you're having a heart attack" application. I've undergone several EKGs, all of which showed nothing was wrong. I have a different program from most people. I can safely override the alarms, concentrate on ignoring the pain and getting on with my life.

Every so often, I suffer another trauma and find myself having to reorganize and rewrite my programs. On December 23, 2008, I fell on black ice when clearing my driveway of snow. For those of you, who haven't heard of black ice, it's clear and makes the black top shiny and dangerous, because it's effectively invisible.

I had an accident in 1996 caused by black ice. We lived in a cul-de-sac, with the exit 100 yards from our house, needing a left-hand turn. The wheel turned easily, but the car didn't, it kept going straight.

Straight wasn't where I needed to go, because that way finished off in a small creek. I let go of the brakes but had no time to finish the maneuver. The car hit the curb and bounced backwards. I got out the car to examine the damage, completely forgetting about the black ice. The result was obvious. As soon as my foot touched the ice, I fell. Unfortunately, I didn't merely slip; I thudded to the ground and pantomimed trying to get back to my feet, falling down several more times. I eventually grabbed the door and dragged myself upright. I hurt my pride and the base of my back. The car fared worse and needed a new front axle.

In 2008, I was clearing the snow off my drive. I cleared the first line across the front of the garage and turned to do the second one. My leg slipped away from under me and the snow was deep enough, according to the surgeon who fixed it, I destroyed my ankle. The loud cracking sound and the sudden agony at the bottom of my left leg made it obvious to me I'd done some real damage. I crawled into the garage, to get some help. There's an old carpet on the garage floor, to help with the fact that in the winter, the concrete gets so cold it hurts to walk on. I wasn't too cold as I dragged my horribly broken body to the garage stairs.

If you're female, you may want to take a short break, so you can stop laughing and wipe your eyes from imagining how wretched I was.

279

It was the day before Christmas Eve and Ann's parents were over to visit. I say over, because we now lived in Utah and our parents still lived in the United Kingdom. They, Ann, some of our married children, our unmarried children and some foster children, are all in the house making a noise. I'm lying pitifully at the bottom of the garage stairs, screaming in a manly way for help. Somehow it managed to sound like a 7-year-old boy, but we won't dwell on that.

Eventually, someone heard the pathetic pleadings coming from the garage and came to investigate. They ran back into the house and got Ann, who looked over the scene and decided to bundle me into the car and take me to the hospital. Unfortunately, I couldn't be bundled. I couldn't stand up; I couldn't take the weight of my body on my wrists to begin standing. I needed to put all my weight on my right foot and there was no way to do so, in the enclosed space I was in, lying there in my pitiable condition. I couldn't crawl up the stairs either, so she called 911.

Put out the fire!

A cop showed up and tried to make me comfortable. A few minutes later, the paramedics arrived, along with a fire truck, presumably in case something needed to be hosed down, or a fire had started. I haven't asked why they do this, yet each of the many times we've called 911 for an ambulance, a fire truck has shown up. I called when Ann had a TIA (a form of stroke) and a fire truck showed up. I had a kidney stone and a fire truck showed up. Oddly, when we called 911 because 14-year-old Amelia was throwing TVs around, no fire truck showed up. Only a sheriff's deputy, a local policeman, a policeman from each of the next two towns and the sheriff. It reminded me of the wonderful album, "Alice's Restaurant." As Ann had had to sit on Amelia to calm her down, this was a time someone needed cooling down with a fire hose.

With the Christmas broken ankle, as soon as I was lifted onto a stretcher, the fire trucks and firefighters left, presumably searching for a fire to put out. In the back of the ambulance, they started hooking me up to machines and stick needles in me, to help with the pain. You'll probably have noticed this contradictory practice, if you've ever had the need to go to hospital for a painful condition. They stick needles in and this hurts. I suppose the idea is to take our mind off the pain, by giving us pain elsewhere. You know, I'll stomp on your foot to help you forget the pain in your arm. It does work for a second, but then you have pain in multiple places.

The ER doctors sent me for X-rays, then straight down to surgery. I had to wait, while they contacted a surgeon who was willing to come in and do the surgery. I was in La-La land, so didn't care. There's a plate on one side and 6 pins on the other. The surgeon told me it was as bad a break as he'd ever seen. Lucky me eh? I have a ground up dead woman and a plate in my left upper arm.

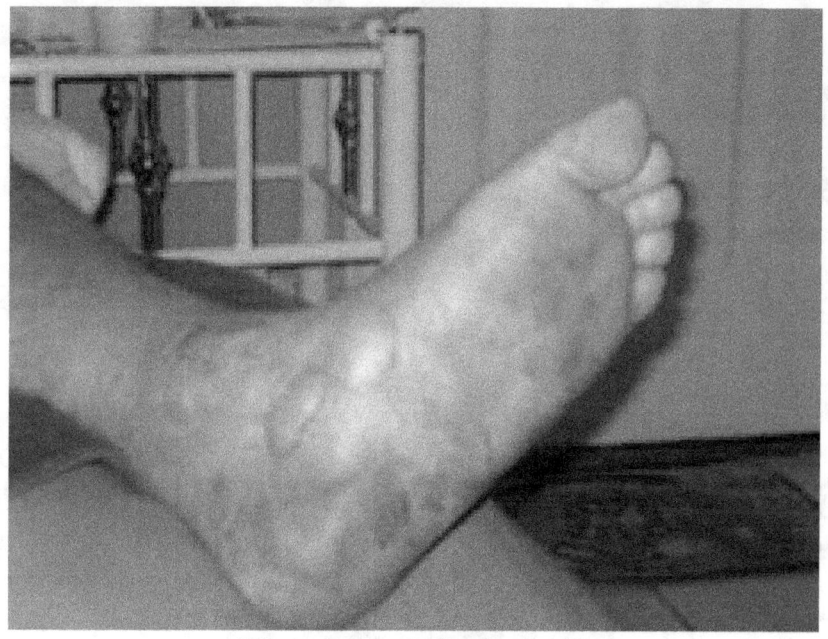

That doesn't look good

The plaster cast was due to come off after two weeks, so the doctor could check the bones and put a walking cast on, if possible. As with all casts, the itching had been horrible and if I tried to move around, the leg swelled up horrendously and my toes turned black. I'd missed most of Christmas, and been stuck in bed since New Year's Day. When the cast came off, I assume the doctor didn't purposely plan to scare me with his comment, "That doesn't look good". The foot and leg were swollen and red. I had huge blisters, from foot to knee. The pads over the surgery sites were soaked solid with blood and covered in yellow gunk.

The doctor suggested I was probably allergic to something they used in the surgery or to the cast materials and wanted me to leave the leg bare, take some more pain pills and come back the next morning. And you thought it was a joke about how it works with doctors. I had no choice but to do so. The leg got worse and worse – hot, a much deeper red, some bigger blisters and much more swollen. The allergic reaction, or whatever it was, had reached my face, which had swollen so much I could hardly see and I was beginning to itch all over my body. We returned to the ER and they prescribed steroid cream, gave me a steroid shot and some antihistamine - super Benadryl the doctor called it. It worked for an hour but then the itching returned. If I stood, the leg and foot turned red. Ann was given a supply of steroids and some needles and told to attack me with them every couple of hours. Each injection site turned black and blue and I had this wonderful multi colored ring around my waist. I'm fairly certain Ann enjoyed "attacking" me. I was glad they stopped me itching and the pain from the ring no longer hurt.

Rotten Dam Syndrome

The places I was already suffering with this Rotten Dam Syndrome (That's dam without an 'n' and yes, I know it spells RDS) were playing up as well. I'd recently found a medication that worked for me with no side effects, except when I forgot to take it. Right now, the medication wasn't working and my left arm was staying at an 8/10 or higher. My back was complaining I was sitting all the time. My neck didn't want to be left out and was hurting. The medication they gave me for the ankle was working a bit. It had some unpleasant side effects, such as constantly burping, constipation and being zoned out, but they made the pain manageable

I couldn't walk. I hurt both arms and wrists to use crutches. I used a walker, but we live in a multi-level house. There are three steps down into the living room from the kitchen. There are stairs into the basement and three stairs down into the craft room and another bedroom. The master suite is upstairs, along a landing and up 3 more stairs. I did a lot of crawling around the house, which hurt as I'd also damaged my left knee and shinbone when I fell. Who needs to call a pity party with all this happening? Well, I do.

The doctor told me it would be months, not days, or weeks, for the ankle to mend and I could walk again. He also suggested the RSD would spread there meaning the pain would never go away. I became quite adept at using a walker during this time.

Curve balls

Our foster children have been in this sort of situation, where no matter what, life seems to get worse. It isn't their fault it simply is! Life seems to throw us curve balls, which, under normal situations, wouldn't happen. Murphy's Law is everywhere and how we handle ourselves when life goes wrong shows the sort of people we are. Our job as foster parents has been to help them realize, their equivalent of the ring of bruises around my lower body, will eventually make life better and the pain and misery they are suffering will eventually go away. The mental pain they suffer is much worse than the problems I suffered from an allergic reaction to iodine.

Not born free, born addicted

Their lives have been ruined by their mother's decisions. They have been forced down paths they didn't want to travel along. None chose to be born addicted to drugs.

When two-year-old Julius came to live with us, he was unintelligible. The experts said he should have been speaking. His mother's methamphetamine use before, during and after the pregnancy, meant he couldn't. For all his short life, before he came to live with us, Julius had been exposed to drugs. A drug test "scored" him at a rate seven times the level where someone is considered a methamphetamine addict. This, along with the lack of parental TLC meant, developmentally, he was between 9 and 15 months.

His three-year-old sister Robyn had a forceful character, which made dealing with her difficult. We quickly realized her "built in" character traits were deciding how she behaved. When they moved into our home and family, we had seven children under ten, along with our 31-year-old son who lived in our basement. Robyn's forceful nature fit in well.

She and Julius began to tag team us. One or both cried constantly from the time they got out of bed. When we have a screamer, all we can do is try to ignore the noise. If they are a baby, we can hug and cuddle them, but eventually we must put them down. We can check they aren't hungry, or dirty, or need something, put them back in their crib and shut the door. Sometimes a closer check can be helpful. A young man I know cried inconsolably when his aunt pinned his manhood to his Terry towel diaper and didn't realize through 30 minutes of screaming.

When your little one follows us around, shouting mom all the time, it can be hard. Especially when we have someone like Julius who called us all mom. He'd follow me around, asking questions and calling me mom every two seconds or so. To make matters worse, he'd often hit me to get my attention. RSD means a soft hit on my left arm feels like a sledgehammer. Naturally, Julius tried to hit me there.

He's DAD not MUM!

Robyn didn't help the situation. She didn't call everyone mom; what she did was keep shouting at Julius, telling him I was Dad. When Julius lived with us, I could easily find Ann in a store. I simply followed the sound of the crying child. He'd cry for something, yet if we gave him it, he'd throw it away. He'd then cry because he didn't have it. No matter how many times we retrieved what he wanted, he

284

immediately threw it away, often at us. At times, getting what he wanted didn't stop his crying, as he wanted to cry anyway.

It took a bit of work, but Julius and Robyn became wonderful children. We got them to a point where they weren't tag teaming us with their screaming. DCFS found some family members who were willing to adopt them and they transitioned from our home to theirs. This couple was wonderful and even traveled the 1200 miles from their house to ours without complaint. The children shifted allegiance from us to them, with little or no issue and even seemed to enjoy the 18-hour journey home.

Our job had been to reprogram their little spirit bubbles, so none of the initial behaviors continued. They may not have suffered physical pain, except with the drug withdrawal but their behavior suggested there was plenty of spiritual, emotional and mental pain to make up for it. The drug withdrawal during those first several weeks, explains why Julius was unhappy, even when he got what he wanted.

We've kept in touch over the years and have loved the updates and the fact they haven't repeated any of those behaviors. They've had many more, but not those. The pain of having them leave us is far outweighed by the joy of knowing they're with loving parents, even though the stork left them at the wrong house. Some of our children, they were left in the wrong country as well. Julius and Robyn were left many hundreds of miles from where they should have been left.

Our spirit bubbles were positively charged, as we knew they were heading somewhere permanent; with people committed to offer them a safe loving home. We were filling our bubbles with service and this made us feel wonderful.

Bugs!

Occasionally, we learn one or more programs our brain automatically runs, is wrong and needs changing.

I was a computer consultant at a bank some years ago, working on a project that took data files from another new project. Unfortunately, the people who were designing the other project didn't check with me regarding something simple. For some insane reason, they decided to store an essential date in a one-character field. They only needed to know which day of the two-week banking schedule it was, I needed to know the actual date. For those of we who aren't computer people, this is disastrous. A one-character field has only 255 possible values. The calendar has 366 possible values. I came up with a solution. Unfortunately, it cost $1 million, in today's money, to fix the error.

Any of the programs we run on the computer systems of our brain could have similar catastrophic bugs. There are thousands of books and tapes available, the purpose of which is to help us rewrite those programs.

For me, the physical body is a mess. I hurt from the top of my head, to the bottom of my feet and all parts in between. I hurt on a scale out of 10, where zero is no pain and 10 is the worst pain, at from 4/10 to 10/10 everywhere. I've written and rewritten my programs over the years, as I've gotten older and hopefully wiser. This rewriting has always been to do with what I can no longer do. Don't run, don't lift more than 10 pounds total, 5 pounds per arm, etc. If I ignore these recommendations I suffer badly. I have also managed to drop whatever it was I was carrying.

No control

Some of our decisions have programmed our brains so the body is in control and our spirit, whether in the captain's chair or not, seem to have no way of overcoming the dangerous programming.

Cigarette smoking is a good example of this. The body craves the nicotine and alarm bells ring, when the level drops. The Ventral Tegmental Area and the Nucleus Accumbens areas of the brain start sounding their alarms, because of the way nicotine affects dopamine. We may try to silence these alarms, but ask a smoker how well they can silence them. I recall seeing a smoker, who had traveled for 8 hours without being able to have a cigarette, lighting three cigarettes and try to smoke them at the same time. He was happy to stand outside even though the weather was atrocious. Millions of people have rewritten the program demanding nicotine and overcome the craving, but until then, they're a slave.

With Julius and Robyn, we'd helped them rewrite the apps so methamphetamine was no longer in control. Life no longer revolved around the horrors the drug withdrawal was causing. They could now run on autopilot and behave like normal 2 and 3-year-old monsters. Just because we'd resolved the problems their mother had caused didn't mean the children wouldn't go through the terrible twos and threes.

We had reprogrammed their brains away from the horror of the drug abuse they suffered.

Reprogramming

Let there be something of a light tone in your life. Let there be fun and happiness, a sense of humor, the capacity to laugh occasionally at things that are funny. (Gordon B. Hinckley)

I haven't slept for more than an hour at a time since March 24, 2002, so my brain is constantly addled, with moments of clarity, all too short. This means I can no longer hold down a job, but I have been able to be a foster parent and adoptive parent. We've adopted four more children since 2002 and fostered a further 50 children.

I **cannot** do anything I want to. It doesn't matter how positive I am, there are limitations caused by the 110+ traumas I've suffered. Most of the time, I don't let this upset me; I acknowledge my limitations and do the best I can within them. This can involve doing nothing more than sitting in front of the television. Occasionally, I even turn it on.

In the same way I didn't choose the path of life I follow, and want to change roads, so our foster children have no control over the path they must follow. Their parents made all the wrong choices and the children suffer the consequences.

The range of abuse our children have suffered is unbelievable and it's been our job to help them get their spirits into the captain's chair and learn how to fill their spirit bubble with joy, despite what has happened to them.

Being positive

Problems can only be solved by being positive. We act as if the things the child is doing don't hurt and accept that we may need to make changes to help them with their pain.

Most of us need to be taught to be positive, but often we're our own teacher. We'd be unable to sit down if we could give the person

288

who causes us the most problems a kick in the pants. In the same way, we'd be hugging ourselves constantly, if we could give the person who can cause us the most good, a cuddle. Being positive is one of the best ways to do ourselves good.

Positive thinking focuses *on the bright side of life* and expects positive results. You Monty Python fans can sing silently here.

A positive person expects joy and happiness, health and success, and believes he or she can overcome any obstacle and difficulty. We may not overcome the obstacle in the way others believe we should, but we should be happy and positive about what we achieved.

Having a positive attitude helps us be happy, **regardless** how life is. I can and do find joy, even though in constant pain. I can help my children be happy, even with the pain they must deal with.

Positivity brings brightness to our eyes and energy and happiness to our whole being. Our spirit can be positive and help us broadcast good will, happiness and success. Even our health benefits from this, we walk tall, our voice is more powerful, and our body language shows the way we feel. I've found people want to be with me when I'm positive, but not when I'm negative. Others are more likely to want to help us if we're positive, but not if our spirit bubble is broadcasting negativeness. This is a problem because it is then we need the most help.

Positivity produces endorphins

Positivity produces endorphins, making us feel good. Begorphins are released when we're negative and they cause more unhappiness and negativity. I don't always succeed but I'm trying to replace pain with discomfort. Pain is a semantically loaded, powerful word, which can make us feel more intensely than using "discomfort". If in our self-talk, we can turn negative ideas or concepts into positive or, at least neutral, ones, we will feel better. Instead of using words such as "hate" and "angry", we can use the words "dislike "and "annoyed" instead because they are softer words.

"I hate this RSD pain condition! It makes me so angry!" becomes "I don't like RSD; it upsets me."

We could make a detailed list of attitudes, thoughts and self-limiting statements, here's a few.

"I can't handle this" or "This is impossible!". These increase stress, but can be turned into positive, hopeful questions such as, "How can I handle this?" or "How is this possible?"

Being positive, gives us power over any circumstance we find ourselves in; instead of the other way around. This is true, even when everything goes pear shaped. I've learned to ignore when others say negative things to and about me and mine, even when they're 100% wrong or 150% if they're American Football coaches who don't understand mathematics. I don't always succeed, but that won't stop me from keeping on trying. I'm the one filling my spirit bubble and I want it filled with positives.

Having been a parent and a husband, through the tough times as well as the good ones, I know how much it's up to me to make everything better. It's up to others as well, but I only control me. I need to be positive so others can follow my lead, because they'll follow my non-positive lead as well.

I can look in the fridge and pantry and find nothing available for me to eat. I'm the only one with Celiac's disease. The cupboards are often full of food I can't eat and empty of what I can. I can complain and whine about this fact OR find something I can eat and stop complaining. Many times, I have to accept this is nothing and carry on without complaint.

Ask my wife how well I'm doing. I plead the fifth. I start the day tired and down. I can fill this page with negativity OR I can put on my big boy underpants and face them down and fill my spirit bubble with positiveness.

I'm tired, because my spirit's using all my resources to fight the pain, leaving nothing much for anything else OR I can celebrate the fact I'm managing and dig deeper for more positivity. I succeed, but I can't say where I get the extra resources from, not because it's a secret, but because I don't know. I simply know I can.

Speak positively

The way we talk forces us to be positive or negative. If we put our head down, slump our shoulders and talk with a complaining, whining tone, we project negativeness. We may have every reason to be negative. We hurt physically, mentally, emotionally or spirituality, or any combination of all four. Or we're depressed about something and on and on.

If, however, we stand up straight with our head and shoulders up, smile and talk with a positive tone, we project positiveness. Forcing ourselves to speak positively makes us feel better. It makes me feel better **EVERY TIME**. I wish I could teach how to force your voice to sound as if you're laughing but I'm not an acting coach. I simply know how to act as if I'm happy and allow my voice to project happiness. If we are projecting positiveness and happiness, we make others happy and positive too. Spirit bubbles become positively charged all around.

We need to speak positively even when we don't believe what we're saying.

This is probably the hardest part of parenting. It's most definitely the hardest part of foster parenting. Many times, I've been grateful a child couldn't see my face, but only hear my voice when I'm praising them. I didn't want to be picking poop out a three-year old's panties. I must calm myself and speak pleasantly about her telling me she has pooped, when I'd preferred she'd gone to the bathroom. This is especially true when we aren't at home and she's already soiled the spare pair of clothing we brought with us. It's even worse when she is three inches from the toilet and she made no attempt to use it.

It's mind bogglingly irritating when a child refuses to eat and behaves as if we're trying to force foul tasting poison down her throat. Especially hard when her mother **has** been starving her and she looks as if she's been in a concentration camp. It is impossible to act rationally and respond in a calm, pleasant voice, but we have no choice. If we want them to begin eating, we learn to bite our tongue, even though it means we get to swallow a lot of our own blood. We must keep telling ourselves it's the amount of food they eat in a forty-eight-hour period that counts and persevere.

When a child has come from an environment where all they've ever received is negativeness, it's amazing to see them begin to blossom, when they realize not all big people are horrible. They begin to believe what we're telling them and forget what they were taught previously. We also communicate positively with our body language, how pleased we are with them. There are consequences for bad behavior, but they are given with love. We positively charge their spirit bubbles for them, in the hope they quickly learn to do it.

How to reprogram

We've been programming, updating and reprogramming our brains since the moment we were conceived. We've continued through to the current day. Our spirit has been allowing our brain to do most of this programming automatically, so we're generally unaware of it occurring. In the same way we use a computer, without knowing how to program it and then later decide to learn how to write programs, we can reprogram our brains.

Here is a list of things that can positively charge our spirit bubble and where we can start with reprogramming.

- *Get as good a night's sleep as we possibly can.*
- *Exercise as much as is possible. I have difficulty but I can move by walking, climbing up and down stairs,*
- *Have an attitude of gratitude. This activates the PFC. Find something you are grateful for. Make up silly things, such as air, if necessary.*
- *Hug the people you love, often. If you only have pets, hug them. If you are like us and have a pet hedgehog, this might not be a great idea. A 20-second hug positively charges even the most negative person's spirit bubble.*
- *Give service*

- *Learn a new hobby and do it often.*
- *Meditate. Even make-belief play charges your bubble.*
- *Deep breathe. The extra oxygen crosses the blood brain barrier and energizes your PFC and therefore our spirit bubble. It gives us the time and ability to concentrate. It also allows us the time to check how positively charged our spirit bubble is and fix it, if necessary.*

The second step in reprogramming our brain is to say what we want. I find it easier to write my goals down before starting, so I don't have to rack my brains to remember. I read the goals aloud. These can be emotional, physical or spiritual. Why out loud? I don't know; I simply know it doesn't work otherwise. There are many things like this in the way in which our brain works. Scientists still have no idea about how the majority of our brains work.

Even though we don't now why, it's a fact that writing down our goals and saying them aloud helps them come true. I suggest that we spend time each day repeating these two steps.

Reticular Activating System

Here's a fascinating brain fact. Our subconscious mind can't distinguish between fact and fantasy. It has no direct links to the outside world. Whatever we tell it, it believes and loads the apps to match those facts. If we tell it we're fat and, even if we're skin and bones, it will set the switches and run the apps we've created for the situation of being fat.

The brain part handling our subconscious behavior is the Reticular Activation System (RAS), which acts a bit like a radio. We are surrounded by radio waves from radio stations and a radio can be tuned to them. Our RAS is programmed to prioritize information, such as listening for particular sounds. We hear our name and all our focus is diverted in the direction we heard it, because that bit of information is tagged as important. The RAS handles one of the strangest abilities we have, the ability not to hear our own 80-decibel snoring, but wake when the baby cries. Another example is when we buy a new car and notice how common it is.

We can use our RAS to cause ourselves problems as well. We can do this with the 'I'm waiting for something to happen then I'll be happy' game. This is when we convince ourselves that everything will be better when we get married or after we are married, we have a child, or another. There is constantly something else over the horizon, we need to happen before we can be happy. Our RAS believes us and ensures our spirit bubble is filled with disappointment when we fail.

When we have children, we are upset when we find that our children are too young and we expect it all to get better when they are older. But they are now teenagers and …. Well, teenagers!

We tell ourselves everything will be better when the house is paid off, we get a better job, a nicer car, when the children get married, when we retire. Then we die and life was not what we wanted it to be. All because we told our spirit, via our RAS that this **is** what we wanted. If this is not what we want, we need to tell our RAS the opposite. We can reprogram our RAS to watch for things related to our goals by performing the steps above.

Have faith in ourselves

The last step is to have faith in ourselves. Believe and expect it all to change. We will all face adversity and challenges, but we need to be sure we don't allow self-doubt or skeptics stop us from overcoming them. Belief is an attitude and nothing can change unless we believe it can. We can choose to believe our spirit bubble can be positively charged and negative emotions released. Or, we can believe the opposite. Our RAS will act accordingly. As always, negative thinking appears to be easier for our RAS to believe, than positive thinking. We must work harder at being positive than at being negative.

Bonding

Ann and I have helped little children reprogram their RAS when their parents haven't merely given the impression they don't love them; they showed them they don't. There is no bond of trust and love

294

between them. All human beings need love and attention; they want to be able to bond to someone. This is supposed to be to their mother and father. It's natural in animals and is shown in the patterning done on newborn animals who think their carers are their parents, even though they're a different species.

The brain's ability to regulate emotions and respond to stress is damaged without bonding. Many children in foster care don't receive this love, attention or bonding. If, by the age of two, a child hasn't bonded to their parents or to another person, it's unlikely they ever will. It's a learned ability and if no one teaches them, before they're much older than two-years-old, it's often too late.

We've found an unloved baby or toddler who hasn't bonded, only needs two or three weeks to learn how to do it. Once they've learned, it's the same as riding a bicycle; we don't forget how. There's no longer any doubt that someone, somewhere genuinely loves them and is willing to give them love, attention, affection, food, clothing and shelter for no reason at all.

There's no hidden agenda, where the adult is only being nice as a prelude, or a postlude, to yet another bout of abuse. They can take this wonderful feeling with them, even if they only received our love and attention for a few months. With all our children, the difference is spectacular. Social workers have joked with us about our special brand of miracle grow. In as little as two weeks, the children change. Happy smiling faces replace the haunted frightened looks they had when they came into care. Elise came to us crying 24/7 and curled into a pretzel shape; she improved after liberal doses of our Tender Loving Care medicine. We've taken babies scared of being touched and helped them look forward to hugs. They've learned how to bond, to give and receive love. This is something no one ever forgets. It's a bit like learning to ride a bicycle, but much more important!

Our secret? It's nothing more complicated than feeding them when they're hungry, changing them when they're dirty, hugging and cuddling them as much as is possible and reasonable and saying positive words to them. The hugging and cuddling are the most important things we can offer any child.

They now have a positive app running, telling them they are worth something; they're not worthless. The negative app has been removed. Knowing somewhere, someone is willing to give us a hug, is one of the most energizing pieces of knowledge any of us can have. It makes us feel wanted, even if only for that moment. Even when it is only short-term, we remember how it felt.

What happens when a child doesn't bond?

Those who don't learn to bond can cause big problems for society Sociopaths cannot bond and are generally amoral. They perceive right and wrong only as it affects them. If doing a thing makes them feel good, it's right, if not it must be bad or wrong.

If they want to do something, it's acceptable even when society may disagree, simply because they want to do it.

Many sociopaths have a superficial charm, but are manipulative and scheming, never recognizing the rights of others. They hide hostility and the fact they are control freaks, below the surface. They lie easily, yet have no feelings of remorse or shame when caught in their lies. In fact, they revel in their lying.

They crave warmth, joy, love and compassion. Their incapacity to give or receive love and their lack of empathy means they use their great acting skills. Their poor behavioral and impulse controls mean they set no personal boundaries, making them irresponsible, cruel and unreliable, all the time appearing to be charming. They are hard to identify and so hard to avoid, even though our own health and happiness needs us to stay as far away from them as we can.

Not all unbonded children become sociopaths

Fortunately for the rest of us, not all un-bonded children are amoral or become sociopaths, but all sociopaths are amoral and have no ability to bond and give or receive love.

Some sociopaths become mass murderers; others become lawyers or work for HMO's (just joking). Although having had to work with a medical system, where health is a cost center and profits are more important than health, especially when the patient is a foster child, I seem to have had to work with too many sociopaths.

If giving warmth, joy, love and compassion to children, reduces the number of sociopaths, we're happy to do our part. We are filling their spirit bubble with joy and at the same time filling our own spirit bubbles with joy as we do so.

If it is to be, it is up to me

Being human, we would expel from our lives sorrow, distress, physical pain, and mental anguish and assure ourselves of continual ease and comfort. But if we closed the doors upon such, we might be evicting our greatest friends and benefactors. Suffering can make saints of people as they learn patience, long-suffering, and self-mastery.   (Spencer W. Kimball)

Can you imagine how great the world would be if we all took the attitude, **if it is to be it is up to me**? That, if something needed doing, **we** did it. This may involve no more effort than talking to the blind person not the guide dog. It may involve talking to the disabled person in a wheelchair, as well as the wheelchair pusher. We have to look beyond the psoriasis, talk to the person and ignore the skin complaint.

We may have to develop a listening ear, so when a friend comes to talk to us about a problem we listen, instead of waiting for them to stop talking, so we can recount the time we had a similar or worse problem. We may have to look beyond the common ideal of only celebrating the winner, so when a family member achieves something, we can praise them for their achievements even though they didn't come first. We don't praise mediocrity, but acknowledge and validate them for what they did achieve and suggest next time they'll do better.

We can donate blood. Say 'bless you' when someone sneezes. Let the other driver have the parking spot. Pick up someone else's trash we find on the street. Thank people for service they give us, even when we're paying them for doing it. Bring joy into the lives of those we meet, by saying something pleasant. We can apologize if we feel we've offended anyone. This can positively charge our spirit bubbles as well as filling other's bubbles with joy.

The list goes on. Each is a simple thing, which, when added together, would make the world so much better than it is. I do them as often as I can and they make my day so much better. As well as adding positively to my spirit bubble, it makes it easier to overcome the pain.

Mirror, mirror

Our spirit bubbles are invisible, but the charge they carry, the emotions inside the bubble are detectable. They show in our body language, especially our face and voice. We can positively charge our bubbles by doing any or all the things on the list. If we want to. This is the master phrase. **If we want to.**

The charge in our spirit bubble is mirrored by those we interact with. Generally, the one with the bigger or higher charge overwhelms the other, lower charged one. This isn't always true, especially when the other person refuses to be overpowered.

A server in a restaurant can bring us out of our funk, because she has learned how to put up barriers to our negativity. She may only be doing this because she knows negatively charged people give little or no tips. Whatever her reasons, it often works. I keep the pain at bay doing it all the time.

Grateful?

Am I grateful for the pain and suffering I've endured? Grateful is the wrong word. My life spiraled onto a new road on March 24, 2002, a road completely different to the one I was on before that date. The original road would have led to riches and no more adopted or foster children. The road I'm on now has led to a lack of money; a number of foster children and four more adopted children.

If I could have an angel pick up the snow pole, so we all got home safely, would I ask it to be picked up so that my life stays on the path it was before the accident occurred?

There seem to be: only two choices available for me to choose from and they are diametrically opposite in their results.

1. Lots of money, no pain, no more children.
2. Lots of pain, little money, foster another 60 children and adopt four of them.

The two are mutually exclusive. Which would you choose? There is no doubt in my mind I'd go for option 2. On that basis, I must say I **am** grateful for being forced to make this choice. I would always choose option 2.

We all have challenges; I'm far from unique in having problems to overcome. What's unique, are my **current** personal trials. No one else has my specific problems. I didn't have them 20 years ago. No one has yours, either. Not one of us has none. All of us have something causing us problems. This is where we need a positive mental attitude and use positive reinforcements.

What have I learned?

Having had all those children, all the broken bones and the constant pain, have I learned anything? I've learned we set artificial limits on what we can do and, at other times, external forces set these limits on us. When we set an artificial limit, we need to get out of our comfort zones and check those limits are valid. This doesn't mean we can do anything and everything we want, that there are no limits to what we can achieve, because there are. There are thousands of books teaching that with the right frame of mind, a positive mental attitude and the will to achieve, we can do anything we want.

I'm sorry but I need to burst that particular bubble; it isn't true. My experience with both pain and children shows me we can't do it all, simply because we want to, or as can occur, someone else believes we should. We should do things only if **we** want to do them, or because it is necessary when we play a specific role. If we do things because someone else thinks we should, or because we think someone else thinks we should, we may find we are doing something we don't want to because we believe someone else should be allowed to make out decisions for us. You may have to read that sentence a few times to see the silliness of it all.

Why run a 4-minute mile

For example, I won't ever run a 4-minute mile. The gurus and experts tell us I'm wrong. I merely need to change my attitude and I'll be able to do it. There are several reasons I won't ever run a mile in less than 4 minutes.

First, is my age. I'm too old to begin the sort of regime necessary to get myself prepared for such a race. The gurus argue it's possible, and I'd have to agree. It's unlikely but possible. At 16, I could run a mile in 5 minutes, so it was possible that, with training, I could have run a sub 4-minute mile. Second, is my weight. I'm 50 pounds overweight. I weighed only 120lbs when Ann and I married. At my heaviest I weighed 249lbs.

Even with the pain medications all causing weight gain and the celiac diet being so high in calories, I could lose the weight. During the six months before Celiac disease was added by my evil fairy godmother, I lost 40 pounds. The pain medications and Celiac's have meant I've put 45 back on.

Third, is the pain I suffer and here is where the whole thing falls to pieces. I physically can't run. The pain in my ankles, hips and back makes it impossible. After running a few feet with my youngest daughter, when her dog pulled the leash from her hand, I had to stop and hobble painfully for a while. I could increase the pain medications, but why would I want to? Trying to run, could cause me a lot of harm because of my ankle.

Roger Bannister didn't simply walk onto a track one day and say, "Today I will run the mile in under four minutes". He had to train hard and work hard to achieve what, in the end, made him world famous. In 1953, the experts said it was impossible to run a mile in less than 4 minutes. The human body was simply not capable of maintaining a speed of 15 mph for 4 minutes. Doctors and physiologists wrote expert papers proving it was impossible for any athlete to achieve this goal. 15Mph was simply too fast.

Bannister chose not to believe the experts and planned to run a mile in less than 4 minutes at a track meet in Oxford on May 6, 1954. To achieve the 4-minute mile, he realized he'd need the help from other athletes in the race and they agreed to help him. They made sure each lap was run within a specific time, with different athletes act as pacemakers. To worldwide acclaim, Banister completed the race in 3 minutes 59.4 seconds. He broke more than a world record; he broke through a self-limiting attitude and proved the experts really are merely drips under pressure.

Within six weeks, Australian John Landy had broken Bannister's world record. Later in the year, at the Vancouver Empire Games, Bannister defeated Landy in a time of 3 minutes 58 seconds. Each year, athletes shave thousandths of a second off the world record, until today high school students can run a mile in under 4 minutes. The current record is below 3 minutes 50 seconds. It doesn't seem likely that it will get much lower, at least that's what the experts keep telling us and the athletes who keep proving them wrong.

How can young men do what was considered impossible 40 years ago? Some of it is to do with better diet and better training regimes, developed over time. They have the ability and now the belief they can, so they do so.

I don't want to run an under 4-minute mile. To use positive terms, it isn't I don't believe I can. It's because I see no benefit to my family or me doing so, especially with the potential further damage I could do, so I don't do it.

We can't do all there is to do in this life

There's much we simply can't commit ourselves to doing, including some that might be on our bucket list.

For me, this includes riding a jet bike across the Snake River canyon. As of 2017, we have five children under 18 at home and Ann and I can't do what others our age, who are empty nesters, can do.

We made the choice when we adopted them. We do wonder whether our peer group friends are right and we're mad. Children, however, don't come with a return policy. I wouldn't want to, even if they did.

Choices

Choices made when younger, limit what's possible when we're older. For example, in later life we may have found we have a talent for music we haven't used. We may not be able to realize our full potential now, especially if we're getting on in years and have many other responsibilities. This doesn't mean we should give up the talent and decide we'll do nothing with it. Possibly all we can do now is to sing in our local church choir. If this is all that is available, do it, celebrate our success and accept we've done all we can, given the past choices we've made. If we can do more, and we want to, do so. The TV talent shows have produced some talented artists who were, by all reckoning, too old to begin a career in the music industry.

Remember, getting older is mandatory, growing up is optional. We don't have to behave like a 60-year-old, because the calendar says we are. I was 60 in 2015 with five children aged 15, 14, 13, 12 and 5 at home, keeping me young. I choose not to act like an old man, although, for some reason, my children will tell you I am one.

As a young woman, Ann didn't get the chance to do much traveling and in some ways regretted the fact. There was nothing she could do, other than be envious when her friends talked about the places they had been, as young adults.

I suggested she took a holiday with my sister and do some traveling with her, while I looked after the children. She couldn't spend months traveling and so she and my sister traveled some 3,000 miles in three weeks touring the Western United States. She couldn't do everything her friends had done, but she did what was possible and now has memories with the same validity as those of her friends. They're also more recent! Interestingly, we now live in the Western United States. Ann can now claim to have done more than her friends ever had the opportunity to do as young adults. The trip filled her spirit bubble with joy and the memory can still positively charge it.

Our roles and responsibilities may well prevent us doing much of what we want to do, so we should do what can be done. For me, pain has limited what I can do but, I try my hardest not to allow this fact bother me too much, too often. As RSD has a deep emotional content, I find myself crying. When I've finished, I square my shoulders, stick my chest out, stand up straight and get on with life. I bring up my

303

shield and refuse to allow negative emotions to stay in, or return to, my spirit bubble. Nature dislikes a vacuum, so positive emotions automatically flow in and positively charge my bubble.

Look at what can be done and do that

We don't have super powers, infinite resources, infinite time, or infinite talents. Don't worry if others believe they could do more, or do better, or we're not trying our hardest. We may need to push ourselves a bit more. You may be the same as me and had to accept the limits are real and others can stick what they think up their left nostrils. This is as true with foster children and those who complain about us bringing "those" children into our home.

Putting our spirits in charge of the control room of our mind and learning how to press the endorphin, serotonin and dopamine buttons is the most important thing I've learned from being a foster parent and from having RSD. We can all cultivate a powerful imagination, and see ourselves in the captain's chair looking young, attractive and suave. Imagine pushing the feel-good buttons. See the pain gates come down and block out the pain until you can manage it. Self-validate and feel better about ourselves, others and the way in which life is for us.

We can tell our younger self, the mental trauma is all in the past, can safely be considered processed and put into its own compartment, where it can sit and rot. This last suggestion may need help from a professional therapist.

Storms

One Sunday, the weather was pleasant enough I commented on my Facebook page about how it was a great start to the week especially for being happy. On the Monday night, Mother Nature again proved her bipolar medicines aren't working. A dry storm blew in, with emphasis on blew, with winds in the 40-mph+ range. The sky turned black, the trees bent, garbage blew around, the cover on our pool ballooned and everything suggested we were in for a soaking. The storm blew and blew and bit like the Big Bad Wolf trying to get the pigs in the brick house, the storm blew itself out.

The storms we go through can feel to us like that. Everything looks dark and depressing; it may feel as if everything is about to be blown away, like the piggy houses made of straw or wood. Occasionally this does happen; a micro-cell storm engulfed me in 2002, leaving my daughter dead and me disabled with constant chronic pain since. So, I know how depressing life can become.

These storms do come into our lives and, like the storm that Monday, bluster and blow, then pass on without doing any real damage. Unfortunately, it's easy to imagine the damage that could be caused and begin to do the worst thing we can do – worry.

Don't just worry!

I don't mean worrying is wrong, unless all we do is worry. If all the first pig had done when the storm came, in the form of the big bad wolf, was worry, as the straw blew away, he would have become the wolf's lunch. He did his best to stand up to the storm, but when all was lost, he saw there was no point in staying and worrying what might happen. He acted, and ran to his brother's house, which was built of sticks. The fairy tale doesn't give details on how he managed to escape; only that he did. The wolf may have been too intent on kicking up the storm, he didn't notice his goal was no longer attainable, the opportunity had passed. It no longer mattered how much he blustered and kicked up a storm, his goal, the pig, was gone. Sound familiar? There was no point in continuing blowing. Nothing was going to help him achieve his lunch goals. It was time to accept this and move on to the next goal – the house of sticks.

The pigs had the same problem at the house of sticks. If all they did was worry, the wolf would have two pork entrées. As the wolf began his one animal tornado impression and the house of sticks fell, the pigs escaped and ran to their brother who had built a house of stone, hoping for safety there.

This time the wolf inspired storm had no effect. Nothing the wolf did had any effect on the house of stone. The foundation was firmer than the straw or stick house and no amount of ranting and railing,

305

huffing and puffing or anything else the wolf tried, had any effect upon the house of stone and the pigs were at last safe. The wolf continued blowing and blustering and the fairy tale has several endings, including one where the wolf climbs down the chimney into a pot of boiling water and the pigs eat **him**.

It's easy to look at the story of the wolf and the three pigs who tried their trotters at house building and see comparisons with how we deal with the storms that come into our lives. Do we worry, or do we do what we can? The key point is the pigs didn't spend much time on worrying, they acted. The wolf also acted and kept on trying, until it was obvious he wouldn't succeed and his goal was no longer achievable. Had he quit when it was obvious he wasn't going to succeed, he wouldn't have been eaten himself. The same is true with our goals, we may have to change our goals. I have a goal of 10,000 steps a day. I couldn't achieve it, so I set a new goal of 7.500 and once I'd achieved that goal I reset it to 10,000 steps. My objective of losing weight is still the same. 10,000 steps is a goal to achieve the objective.

Our RAS believes us!

Remember, our RAS has no link to anything outside the brain, it believes what we tell it. When we tell it we must pay a bill in the morning, but have no money to pay it, and we should spend the night trying to solve the problem, it doesn't care the problem is unsolvable. It only cares it needs solving and will keep us awake trying to solve it.

So, as the song says, don't worry, be happy. Now, assuming you know the song, you have something to worry about. How to get rid of the ear-worm singing the song. The tried and tested way is to go to YouTube and play the entire song. Off you go! That's where I'm headed! It's a great song and will fill our spirit bubbles with good emotions.

Accept what we can't do, celebrate what we can.

I've come to recognize I have some limits, not present at 3:04pm on Sunday, March 24, 2002.

I've had enough subsequent mishaps to learn my limits keep changing and continually inwards, constantly less. There will always be days when I can't cope and I must admit those days are lost. There are also days when I can cope and those days I celebrate. I accept what I can't do, with the least amount of complaining I can and celebrate what I can do. I have as positive an outlook as I can. I find joy and happiness wherever they may be hiding. I smile even when I want to cry. As my RAS does what I ask it to do, my spirit bubble is full of joy and happiness.

Recognize my limits

The hardest part has been learning to recognize my limits and not put unnecessary stress on my body. I can't lift more than 10 pounds at a time. If I do, the pain in my wrists, arms, neck, shoulders and back skyrocket. What do I do? I split the weight of the object, so I can lift it, or I ask someone else to help. With my babies, I accept the pain will skyrocket and deal with it. My babies are worth it, a 56lb bag of potatoes isn't, unless someone else isn't available to do it. I then simply suffer the increased discomfort and hope I can speedily get it back down to a manageable level. With only three children married, we're already at nine grandchildren. With the other five living ones, this number will get much higher and I'll be picking up babies for some time to come.

Learn to accept the obvious

One of the hardest things any of us has to do is to accept when we're wrong especially when that involves us doing things differently. For a while, the wolf appeared to be having some success with his one animal storm. Appeared to being the key word, he only appeared to be succeeding. He wasn't, because his goal was lunch and what he actually did was blow two houses down.

When what we're doing isn't providing the results we need we must change what we're doing. Albert Einstein is generally credited with the statement, "**Insanity: doing the same thing over and over again and expecting different results.**"

The wolf would have died of starvation if all he did was blow houses down. The fairy story generally has him climbing down the chimney instead, once it was obvious he didn't have the huff and the puff to blow the brick house down.

The straw and wood house pigs hopefully didn't rebuild using the same materials.

I have many obvious things I have to accept because of RSD, Celiac's disease, Opioid Induced Constipation (OIC), etc etc. I could make a very long list of things I can no longer do, which prevent me from doing fun things.

There is no point worrying or stressing about these self-evident issues as they will drive us mad. We have to find work-arounds and if there is none then we must accept it is not possible.

Having had at least one handicapped child since I began parenting, I know how hard it is to accept handicaps, both in my children and myself. My oldest son, now 38, tells me he is happy to accept his handicaps as all the good things that happened because he was handicapped wouldn't have happened otherwise.

I also know parents who refused to accept their child was handicapped despite all evidence to the opposite. I also know of parents who handicapped their children with their overpowering interference. If your child cannot walk or talk; it is insane to keep pushing them to behave as non-handicapped children. Accept the obvious and concentrate on what they can do instead. Put all your energy into that and your child will have the best life possible. Refusing to accept the obvious, both for ourselves and our children can only fill everybody's spirit bubble with massive amounts of negativity.

Parenting – a permanent role

Ann has been pregnant five times and we have three biological children, Simon, Andrew and Amy. We use the term biological, or bio, to show Ann and I are the physical, genetic, biological mother and father. Ann carried them in her womb and gave birth to them. They have been with us since they were born. Even though all three have married and moved away, they're our children and will be forever. Being a parent is a role we always have. As they've grown up, Ann and I have found our parental roles have altered with relation to them. We may no longer have total day to day responsibility, but we are still their parents and always will be. The responsibilities have also increased.

Now, we go to sandwich shops and buy sandwiches I can't eat, because I have Celiac's disease, and sit and watch my married children and their spouses and children eat them. In the past, I ate along with them. Why do I do this? I'm their dad and granddad. That's it. Simple and uncomplicated. I'm their dad and granddad and am happy to play these roles

I celebrate being a father

Our foster children have come into our lives when one or both parents broke the rules and put their children in danger. As well as the children we've fostered, there have been many waifs and strays who have lived with us, when they have apparently crossed a line at home. Some children have found themselves kicked out the family home shortly after their eighteenth birthday, because their parents believed their responsibility ended as soon as the child became an adult. They've found themselves needing somewhere to live and have shown up at our door, at various times of the day, even in the middle of the night. We have always welcomed them in.

Some fit the criteria for being abused, but it wasn't reported. They all have a horrible problem few parents can deal with. It can turn a wonderful, helpful, sweet child into a monster, who wants nothing to do with us; I'm referring to the disease of puberty, or being a teenager.

Ann and I have often suggested we should put a sign above our door like the one on the Statue of Liberty. Engraved on a plaque on the base of the statue is the poem "New Colossus" written by Emma Lazarus. The last part reads:

Give me your tired, your poor,
Your huddled masses yearning to breathe free,

309

The wretched refuse of your teeming shore.
Send these, the homeless, tempest-tossed, to me:
I lift my lamp beside the golden door.

We are a refuge

The many young people, who've beaten a path to our door, have come looking for affection and care, or somewhere to stay, until they'd sorted out their problems at home. We haven't counted these waifs and strays in our 130+ children, because we've no clear idea how many there have been. Some have stayed overnight and others for weeks or months. Some have returned many times. All have stayed with us for as long as they needed to. We've kept in contact with some as they have grown up, married and had children themselves.

Our home is a refuge where our children, grandchildren and occasionally random children from the neighborhood can find safety, love and care.

David Alan Gray

Fill That Bubble

Happiness for me is to know that my life has meaning and purpose, and that every day my life touches others in a positive way – whether to make them laugh or learn or both at once! (Deanna Mascle.)

Each of us starts the day by getting out of bed and choosing how the day will go, based upon on where we are starting from. We can decide the day will be good, or we can expect the day to be horrible. This is where we have control.

I have no control over pain or having had a good night's rest. Nighttime brings little sleep and a lot of pain and discomfort. Lying on my back, sides or front hurts, making it impossible to get comfortable enough to stay asleep, I celebrate what sleep I do get and decide to get on with life anyway. This only changes my attitude, which is all I have any control of. I decide each new day will be wonderful and magnificent. This doesn't guarantee things won't go wrong today, but my bubble is full of positivity.

You must have noticed how, even when we expect the day to be good, life can happen to make it hard. We are as positive as it's possible to be. Our spirit bubble is filled to brimming with optimism and upbeat emotions; anyone coming close to us feels better. Then life happens and throws too much at us in quick succession. We begin to lose our upbeat attitude. At other times, we spend too much time with people whose spirit bubbles are full of negative emotions, who are unenthusiastic and have bad attitudes.

Regardless of how wonderful I know the day will be, life can still be hard to manage. I can put on my depressed hat and whine there's nothing to be positive about. People are being so difficult that it is hard to keep calm and not lose our temper. This is especially true when the other person is losing their temper with us and we cannot understand why they are so upset.

Humor positively charges my spirit bubble

Alternatively, I could tell you my six-year-old daughter recently asked me if, when our pet hedgehog dies, could we keep the body and use it as a brush? That is accepting **it is what it is**, in this case a dead hedgehog, and finding a way to make it useful.

Or, I could tell the story of the thief in South Africa, who saw a car at a set of traffic lights, with the roof down. On the passenger seat was a large bag and the thief thought it would be easy to run over, snatch the bag and get away, before the driver could react. He was correct and got clean away with the bag. What he didn't know was the driver was a professional snake catcher, who had recently been on a job to a local house, which had been invaded by a huge black mamba, the world's deadliest snake. Poetic justice, especially if he put his hand in the bag, before checking what was in it.

Humor relieves the stress from when our spirit bubble is under attack from other people's negativeness. I can also negatively charge my spirit bubble from the inside. For example, as I sit here with a few hundred words written today, I'm feeling depressed, dejected and down in the dumps. I have a lot to be depressed about and … OR as I sit here, having written several hundred words, I choose to be in good spirits. The same number of words has been written whichever way you look at it.

It is what it is. How I deal with it matters.

I may have to force myself to be cheerful and joyful, happy and joyous, but I decide who I am. Am I a person with pain so bad it cannot be overcome? Or am I a person with that same horrible pain, who believes it can be managed? I have decided I cannot surrender to the constant chronic pain; I must deal with it. The same is true as I deal with the many miserable, heartbreaking and distressing events constantly occurring in my life. It's also true, if there is nothing but wonderful, positive, upbeat events happening. I choose to be optimistic because there is no other sensible choice. I also choose to apologize when I have failed to stay positive and upbeat. This is very important as it shows that I am a person who is willing to accept I am not perfect and sometimes get it wrong.

The pain is a constant.

If I wanted to, I can easily give in to the pain. I could ask my doctor for pain pills that will take all the pain away and accept they take my brain with them. I could then vegetate in front of the TV all day, in a medication induced fog. I choose not to do this, because I have a wife, nine children, five who still live at home. I also have 3 married children and 9 grandchildren. They all need me to be capable and available. In 2017, I played the role of big brother, when my younger sister's 24-year-old son died of tonsillitis. This is such a unique situation it was hard to come to terms with. We were all positive and, the whole week I was in Switzerland, we all did our utmost to have positively charged spirit bubbles, even during the funeral and the burial.

I __will__ be joyful!

I choose to be in good spirits. I **will** be as cheerful and joyful as I can, **regardless** of what is happening in the world inside and outside of me. Even when I'm dealing with trauma as preposterous as my 24-year-old nephew dying from something such as tonsillitis, I can find joy. I had the opportunity to spend some time with my mother and two sisters for a few days. Preposterous was my nephew's favorite term and what happened to him can only be defined as such.

When I took inventory of my life, I decided being a husband and a father were the most important roles I play and the ones I would give as much of my disposable time as I could. These roles easily fit within the idea of **"it is what it is"** because, once I married Ann, I was a husband and, once our first child was born, I became a father. There was nothing I could to do to stop these roles and their associated responsibilities automatically becoming mine. I wouldn't want to stop. I know for some people that the result of their actions makes them a parent this is an unwanted intrusion into their lives. It doesn't matter what they think, they are a parent.

Use disposable time on what is important.

Disposable time is the time during the day I have control over. It's the time left over after I have done what I **must** do, such as work, pay bills, etc. I don't have time to wallow in self-pity at the same time as go to the doctors with my daughter. I cannot sit around feeling unhappy and be taking another to volleyball practice or watch her play in her games. I know I **can**, I know it's possible, but nobody would enjoy my presence. If I complain, it becomes obvious I don't want to be there and this isn't what I want to have believed.

My goal is to use my disposable time doing what I can with my family, as best I can. I accept I **cannot** do much of what I used to, but I can do what is most important to me, the best I can.

So, who am I?

A question I ask myself a lot is who am I? For me, life stays hard. Even if I didn't have the problems besetting me with the house, my children and their families, my grandchildren, with money, or the lack of it, I still live in a world of chronic physical pain and discomfort. I can't seem to get people to come to my website. I can't get people to go to Amazon and buy my books. …. Okay, I'd better stop or I will bore you and upset me. This negative thinking waits to pounce as soon as we let our guard down.

One quick and easy way to find who you are is to work out what defines you. If you can, take a time diary. This requires us to be honest about what we are spending our time on. If we keep one for a week, we will be able to see what we spend our time on. According to some statistics, teenagers have approximately 9 to 11 hours screen time a day. They then spend an extra 2 hours texting. That works out at 84 hours a week and would define a teenagers most important role is cell phone user. Whatever we spend the most time on, is the most important thing in our lives. This defines us. Not pains, not trials. It is what we spend the most time on. I spend the majority of my time as a father and husband, so that defines me.

The other part of defining myself is what sort of father, husband, etc am I? Am I a quitter, a defeatist? Or, positive, cheerful, optimistic and joyous? We can have an attitude of gratitude, or of a constant complainer. The choice is ours. We choose to fill our spirit bubble with either positive or negative emotions.

I will use the **"act as if"** method and **act as if** life wasn't bad. My life is what it is, and I must live it, whether it's good or bad. I will be positive and accept things are what they are without needing any adjectives at all. They may not be wonderful and amazing, nor horrible and dreadful. They could be totally mundane, somewhat boring and completely normal.

It would be so easy to allow my spirit bubble to be overwhelmed by all the negativism from those around me. But I refuse to let it. I'll be the positive person, projecting positiveness from my spirit bubble and overpowering their negative ones. Someone must do it, why not me?

Our sports team won or lost, even if we're unhappy with the result. Our attitude has no effect on them. We can't affect most of what happens to us, as most of life continues with or without our input. The things that happened in the past are also outside of out of control. There isn't even a replay button so we can be sure we remember it correctly.

Final score – us 0, them 10

Our reaction will not change the fact the soccer team you played on lost 10-0 in the final of the competition, as happened to a team I was on, back in 1969. I still remember our goalie's response at half time when we were losing 5v0; he took off his lucky charm and disgustedly threw it away.

On a positive note, I recall the fun of being on the team and remember with joy, we were playing in the competition finals, against a team where the youngest member of their team, was older than the oldest player on our team. We'd won all the games leading up to the final and I can happily recall those memories. The score was still 0 –

10 in the final and nothing will change that. Years later it's as fixed as in 1969. Nothing can change that.

I can affect what's happening now, but things may still go pear shaped. As I wrote this line, my daughter called from school and asked me to bring her a pain pill. I can rant and rave about the interruption, or I can be happy I have a 16-year-old daughter, who needs her daddy's help and be the sort of dad who will immediately go help her. I chose to be that sort of dad because my daughter is very important to me. I cannot think of anything else I could have done for that half hour that was more importantly than going to the school that morning.

Laugh about it and act as if people aren't nasty

When my chair fell over on the beach during the summer, I made light of what had happened and lay there while my family took pictures. I can now laugh about it and have the picture to prove what happened.

Nothing will change the fact I have RSD, so I accept and manage it. Each day begins the same way and I cajole, coerce and generally force myself to feel good. I can and do inject joy into the way I speak, not necessarily talking the way I feel.

When my 3-year-old granddaughter pulled the blinds down in the living room, and I mean down as in off the wall, I made a joke of it and simply put them back up. I've learned shouting at a child over this sort of thing, doesn't change the fact the blinds are lying in a heap on the floor, nor put them back in front of the window. The only way to save me from blindness, because the blinds weren't up and blocking the blinding sun, was for me to stand on the sofa and put them back, so they could serve the purpose for which they were created. I believe you'll find this blindingly obvious.

We can all act "as if" the people in our life are **not** being unpleasant and pretend their behavior is not a personal attack on us. We do what's possible without worry, complaint or concern.

316

Having read some of what I've dealt with, you might think you want to swap your problems for mine, although I doubt it. I'm positive, however, I don't want yours.

Grateful?

Am I grateful? I am. I wish the pain would go away, instead of getting worse, but wishing changes nothing. Anyway, I may not be able to handle whatever replaces that challenge. Nature abhors a vacuum so you can guarantee something else will come along. I can work with my personal trials and find joy, happiness and fulfillment in living, joy in serving my family and others, even joy when my favorite sport team loses, again!

Our children are growing up. Three are married and have given us 9 grandchildren. The rest are still at home. Regardless of how crappy I feel. It doesn't matter I feel as if I have the flu 24/7 or I get little or no sleep. Who cares if (and only I can say this) 90% of my body is feeling pain, at 9/10 or higher, has done so for some time and will do so for the foreseeable future? Or that I'm permanently tired? What matters is my family. For my wife, I will be there all the time. I'll be here, being a dad, until my children no longer need me to be there for them all the time. Then I'll be there for my grandchildren and great grandchildren. I'll find joy in the pain and ensure I spread joy and happiness wherever I am, especially to and with my family. My spirit bubble will remain positively charged.

The world may well be falling to pieces around me, but I will still be happy, and joyful. The world may well be headed to hell in a hand basket, wherever this place called hell is and how we'd get the world in a hand basket anyway; I will still be joyful and positive.

Every day brings something new.

One thing 130+ children have taught me is that, while you'd think I'd know it all, I don't. Every new day brings something new to deal with, new problems to overcome and new reasons to smile sweetly and ask my 6-year-old to stop jumping on my back.

317

If I must suffer through grief and catastrophe as well, I admit I'd prefer not to, but bring that on as well. I'll find joy anyway, even through pain, misfortune and calamity. My spirit bubble will continue to be positively charged to overwhelm any negativeness.

At our peak and copacetic

We should act as if we are at our peak and whatever is happening will not get us down. Even though life, the universe, the gremlins or whatever is giving us grief and making our day miserable, it's important, in fact essential, we act as if everything is copacetic. I love this word, I can see 1960s flower power people using it. It means everything is satisfactory and acceptable. It's a state of mind that says, "You know what? I'm going to be happy, regardless of what's happening."

Copacetic may have a different meaning to me, than it means to you. A good day for me, may be a totally horrible one for you.

Copacetic days for you could be unacceptable to me and negatively charge my spirit bubble. We all respond differently and what's easy for one to handle may be completely impossible for someone else to deal with.

Copacetic is a completely personal concept. If it's satisfactory to you, it doesn't matter what others think or feel. It is important that you find a way for life to be copacetic for **you**. Live within **your** moral boundaries, give service and fill your spirit bubble with joy and you will be copacetic.

Copacetic means not complaining.

There are a number of words meaning the opposite of copacetic including unsatisfactory. When we find very everything is unsatisfactory, I'm sure you realize that the best word to describe what we do is **complain.** The list of synonyms of complain is quite impressive –

beef, bellyache, bitch, bleat, carp, caterwaul, crab, croak, fuss, gripe, grizzle, grouch, grouse, growl, grumble, grump, holler, inveigh, keen, kick, kvetch, moan, murmur, mutter, nag, repine, scream, squawk, squeal, wail, whimper, whine, yammer, yawp, yowl, protest, quarrel (with); cavil, quibble; fret, stew, worry; blubber, cry, sob; bemoan, bewail, deplore, lament.

An interesting list that I would have to call you mendacious if you claim never to have been "guilty" of many of those words. If you don't know the word mendacious, sorry.

To be totally copacetic we need to give up complaining. Sounds easy, I know. When we talked about complaining, I said we may need to complain; like when the food is poor quality. That is using the second definition of complain – making a complaint. I am talking solely about the moaning type of complaint.

As I said, a hard objective. Hard enough that I haven't fully achieved it myself. I have a lot of things to complain about.

At the beginning I had the goal of not complaining for the first hour after getting out of bed. I also want to not complain in my head, as well as out loud. I am still working on it. I am also still working on not complaining to or about others, but I will keep on trying. I **will** replace the negative in my spirit bubble with positive feelings.

So... What?

To make everything copacetic I need to use the principle of **"So... What"**. Not so what? I don't care. It means, **so** this situation exists and it needs to be changed, **what** am I going to do to change it? So I'm not 'being there' for my children much as I'd like to be, what am I going to do about it? I can then set some goals and targets so that am. What I can't do is simply give up. The same is true of you. What has happened up to this point happened in the past, all we can do is make a difference in the future. There's no such time as too late.

I'm never going to be there for my children all the time. They may be a priority, but the other roles and responsibilities I've accepted will mean I have to do other things as well. For example, I need to go to work to provide for their physical welfare. I have a wife and it is important that we spend time without our children, just us two. I have to give myself some time as well. The chunk of time left over is what I give to my children.

So, I'm not there for my spouse? What am I going to begin doing right now to fix that problem? Not, what do I need to get our spouse to change? What **do I** need to do? We need to always be there for our spouse and ensure love never speaks evil. Once the children are gone, all that's left is the two of you. Our spirit bubbles will have to be operating together and we will both need to be fighting any pain, whether physical, spiritual, mental or emotional or any combination of them. Ann and I will be old by the time LLO9 flies the nest in the next 15 or so years. For most of us, this occurs when we are middle aged. I say most of us because Ann and I may never be empty nesters. If we are not "there" for our spouse now, how can we be there for them in the future?

There's a simple principle, hard to put into practice but easy to talk about. The best way to deal with people, who aren't doing what we would like them to, is to act as if they are. We can't always change the behavior of others immediately, but we can control ours and the idea that love thinks no evil, allows us to behave as if the other person is already changing. All the literature on this topic reports that the other person will respond by changing. If our spirit bubble stays positive in relation to our spouse then use the simple rule of the spirit bubble with the stronger emotions will overpower the one with the weaker emotions. A negative attitude to our family member is dangerous because our spirit bubble could overpower everyone else's.

Fighting Pain Finding Joy among chaos

My motto is *fight pain find joy*, but I know how easy it is to be finding pain and fighting joy. Some people don't seem to want their lives to be copacetic.

In many families, the parents and the children seem intent on using the law of entropy in all of their dealings with each other. The law of entropy means everything breaks eventually and the normal state for most things is chaos. A phone wire is a prime example. Put one in a drawer and try to remove it a few minutes later.

There are many examples from life that prove chaos rules. Here are a few simple equations.

- *Take a tidy room, add a child of any age, and we get a messy room. Tidy the room and chaos and entropy will rule immediately after the child returns.*

- *Add car tires to a stony, bumpy, pot holed road we will quite possibly get a flat tire. Or, as I found out a short time ago, five flat tires.*

- *Add caffeinated soda to a child we will get a crazy creature. I love the sign I have seen in many stores that reads, "Unattended children will be given a caffeinated soda and a free puppy."*

- *Two 3-year-olds plus a toy, any toy equals fight.*

- *Teenager plus a gaming computer equals a brainless organism, occasionally a full-blown zombie.*

- *Teenager plus chores equals sickness.*

- *Teenage daughter plus dad plus mall = broke dad.*

Then there are the equations we have to deal with as spouses. A husband knows when there are two choices, his wife will tell him he chose poorly, regardless of what he selects. If he could rewind time and choose the other option, she'd still tell him he is wrong. This is especially true when she asks him to select which shoe looks best or what top goes best with the skirt she has selected. Or the most dangerous choice of all, "Does this make me look fat?"

As a wife, you will live in a different time dimension from your husband. The time between your husband agreeing to fix something and it being fixed is a short time for him and a long time for you.

When we need a child to make a choice, it is best to suggest the option we don't want them to make. That way, we can guarantee they'll make the choice we want them to. This may work with your wife as well.

The last one is the law that says if it's broken and we try to fix it to save money, we'll make things worse and it will cost twice as much to fix as the original estimate. More things will also need fixing. These "equation" are funny to talk about, but they are all experiences where those involved could be upset, or at least annoyed. With each, it can be very easy to fight the joy and find the pain.

Don't fight the joy

I've had many experiences where I could have easily fought the joy, but I decided to find the joy, even when it actually involved pain for me. One happened one Friday, as I was painting the kitchen table. We'd decided it was time to have a new color and I was painting the table with white primer. My daughter wanted to help, so she found a little artist brush and started to paint with me. Unfortunately, she managed to leave paint drops all over the kitchen floor. I also had to paint over the unwanted blobs on the table she left. It took me an extra hour to clean up the mess she had made, most of it on my hands and knees with a paint scraper.

As well as being annoying it also seriously hurt. An able bodied person would have taken 15 minutes to clean up. It took me an hour. I was not feeling particularly copacetic, but my daughter, hopefully, has absolutely no idea of this and she will not recognize herself or that I was upset.

Should I be upset?

I chose not to be upset! I want her to have good memories of helping dad. I want her to find joy in the memory and be able to say she helped paint the table. I don't want her to have painful memories and remember me shouting and complaining about the mess she'd made. As the laws of the universe make sure we remember the bad things before the good things, had I shouted and complained, instead of just cleaning the mess up quietly, she'd remember being reprimanded the next time she saw me painting. This is a major part of being a parent. We can't allow ourselves to be upset, for our children's sake.

Shouting disproves that love thinks no evil

I make an effort, which means I don't always succeed, to avoid shouting at my children, even when they need to be shouted at, especially then. It takes a lot of self-control not to shout when this is the third time in the past few minutes we've asked them to do or not do something. I know from personal experience I've created some painful memories for my family, which I really want to able change to joyful ones. All I need is a time machine and a note saying "Don't shout, it's not that important! Remember love thinks no evil." Only then will I, possibly be able to learn to not shout at my children. Hopefully sooner than later.

I joke that the only one of my children who doesn't cause me this pain is my second daughter, Elizabeth, and that is because she died in 2002. This dark humor isn't true, because I miss her. She'd have been 26 in 2017 and used to joke she wasn't leaving home until she was 23. We never have to look far to find pain and fight joy and need to force ourselves to fight the pain and find joy. If not, pain will win and joy will be forced from your spirit bubble leaving you with a negatively charged spirit bubble.

Adult children generally don't cause the same level of pain as teenage children. This is because they have matured sufficiently and, of course, have their own children to deal with. The major reason things are easier with our married children is that they have moved out of the family home and we don't see them all the time. It's the same reason grandchildren are considered to be better than children. We can send them home to their parents, sometimes with a caffeinated drink.

Being copacetic with my children

As I want everything to be copacetic, I can, at least, make sure I am causing as little pain with and to my family. I can also do all I can to find joy and share it with them.

With our children, especially when they are teenagers, we can often feel we are on the beaches of Dunkirk when all we want is to know is how they did at school. This is when we double down, or deca-down or however many levels it takes and ensure we only find joy and fight the pain. I'm an optimist, I believe that showing love thinks no evil means, eventually, I will receive no evil back. My 3rd child, our oldest daughter sent me a Facebook message when she was 25 and had 2 children. It said, "You were right all along, David Gray." This filled my spirit bubble with joy when I read it and still does.

Knowing who my children are.

After our first three children were grown and married, we still had 5 adopted children at home. In fact, we still do right now. With all our children, we've had to get to know who they were.

Many parents claim to be surprised by what their children have done, having no idea of their abilities, talents and interests. Not too surprisingly, these children don't show any interest in their parents once they've grown up and left home. Pop star Harry Chapin wrote the song "The Cats in the Cradle" about a father who never had time for his son as his son grew up. When the son left home and never wanted to visit, he'd give the same excuse his father had. I have to believe both of their spirit bubbles were negatively charged when they thought of each other and how the other person was rude and cruel.

Getting to know our children takes time. It involves taking the high road and scheduling time to do things with them. Things they want to do, not necessarily things we want to. Researchers have identified that the average parent spends about an hour a day with their children, sometimes as little as 6 minutes, a day talking with them!

I spend a lot more time with my children and with my wife than this, because I've decided they're very important to me. I believe giving of that most precious of resource, time, to my children will show them I love them much more than any physical gift, toy etc. can ever do.

Children have their own feelings, ideas and attitudes. When we get to know what they're feeling, what their beliefs and standards are, we get to know them better and, more importantly, they know they're loved. Making time for our children involves sharing experiences with them – being happy when they are happy and sad when they are sad. It involves teaching them we take them seriously and that what they are saying and doing matters. I've learned to mute the TV when I'm talking to them and to look them in the eye as I do so. I want to watch the show or the movie, but the high road, showing my children I believe love thinks no evil requires me to do so. When I'm writing I'll swing my chair around from the keyboard and screen to give them my attention. I want our spirit bubbles filled with joy, and pain to be as little as possible.

Am I an expert at this? Would my children find my behavior copacetic? I know that my wife does not always, because I often fail to give her 100% of my attention. I'm working on it though. She may not find my behavior un-copacetic and argue I'm on the low road, failing to show love. I obviously would argue otherwise, but I'd also have to agree I'm not always being there for her.

This is me admitting to you I'm falling short. This is also me telling you that by the time you get to read this, I'll have resolved the issue and it will no longer be a problem for me.

Being there for our spouse and children

I've come up with a list of things that define how I can show I'm there for my family. Here, in no particular order, is that list.

- *Being there for them means taking the time to listen to their concerns. It means knowing them well enough to be able to help them with their problems. It means remembering that listening involves two ears and one mouth. It is very easy for us to give them advice when all they want is for us to listen and validate their feelings. They often don't want any advice, they know what to do and just want to talk about it.*

- *It means encouraging our children to come to us with their problems and questions. Having a listening ear, a loving heart and helping them solve their problems if we can and they want us to help solve it. It means not being impatient when they ask questions or need some time. It means validating their right to be upset with what's going wrong.*

- *It means attending the school concert, play, or sport games. Children can be a pleasure to be with one moment and embarrassing the next, especially when taking part in school activities.*

- *It means not getting upset or annoyed if they make a mistake and always trying to compliment them on how they did; even if they didn't do well.*

- *It means coming home from work and spending time with them instead of with the work we have brought home.*

- *It means creating once in a lifetime experiences.*

- *It means helping them with their homework and other projects, and not belittling their efforts.*

- *It means being the parent we always wished we could be.*

- *It means loving them unconditionally.*

- *It means letting them make their own decisions*

When I look at the list, I worry I'm not doing well with the items on the list with my own children. I can make the list and show what I should be doing but realize that I'm not yet achieving everything. This doesn't mean I'm not trying, nor does it prevent me from suggesting it to others. It means I've not yet achieved the goal of being as good a father as I want to, but I'm going to keep on trying. My spirit bubble may not always be positive; I may be in a huge amount of pain and finding it hard to positive my spirit bubble. I will keep on trying.

This list is valid for the one more important than my children or anyone else in my world, my wife. I know how, when life is spiraling out of control, we can temporarily forget this fact. It's very important we do all we can to always be there for our spouse and that this relationship is always copacetic. To do this, we must fight any pain we suffer and find joy in our marriage regardless of what our experiences may tell us.

So, what else have I learned?

There are many things I have learned over my life especially from having had 130+ children and suffering chronic whole body pain. As we have traveled together in this book, I hope you have been able to identify them. Here are a few from my own plan of happiness. They're mine and I'm not suggesting you should use them yourself. Well, I am, but you don't have to.

Rules

In order to to achieve anything in life we need to have a rule set by which we live our lives and by which we help our children learn to live their lives in a productive manner.

These rules need to be age and situation appropriate. Currently, I have 5 distinct types of house rules. One each for (1) my married adult children; (2) for my teenage children; (3) for my young children; (4) for my grandchildren; (5) for guests. I have different rule sets I use in different public places, such as at a movie house; a theater; at church; or in a store. We have the rules of the road and the rules of the society we are parts of and there are rules such as the Ten Commandments.

A life lived with no rules will eventually produce a society without any.

Direction

The direction we are heading in and with our lives are determined by the rules we follow. Our morals and values such as honest, patience and respect make us who we are.

With our children, we need to show them guidance. direction, and help with their morals and values. We can't expect the schools to do this, because we may find they are taught morals and values we don't agree with,

Goals

Very little in life is accomplished without goals. We may have rules and know the direction we are headed, but without goals we will not keep headed the right way.

As failing to achieve a goal is a guaranteed way to fill a spirit bubble with negativity and with pain limiting my abilities, I must set realistic goals, ones I can achieve. I do this regardless of how much I hurt, hopefully showing how it builds character and compassion. Victor Franklin said, "In some way, suffering ceases to be suffering at the moment it finds a meaning."

Biological needs

We need to take care of our own basic biological needs such as food, water, shelter, somewhere to sleep, medical needs and clothing. If we have children, it is our responsibility to do the same for them. We must be running at peak efficiency, to be able to do this. For me, peak is more like a valley, so, I take naps and do less of what **I** want to do, and do whatever it takes to keep my spirit bubble full of joy and happiness. My children feed off my bubble, so I must have a positively charged bubble so they can.

Loving others, especially our children

C.S. Lewis put it well "The Christian doesn't think God will love us because we are good, but that God will make us good because He loves us." Foster children have often been shown their parents do not love them. Our job has been to fill their spirit bubbles with joy by showing them **we** love them.

Encouragement

With children we should encourage them, give them lots of affection. They will grow and their spirit bubbles will fill with joy, in part because they want us to keep encouraging them.

With us, especially when we are in pain, we need to encourage ourselves to be positive, and keep our spirit bubbles positively charged. This is true in our relationship with other people as well. Remember the spirit bubble with the strongest emotion overwhelms the weaker one. We need to encourage others as often as we can.

Education

Education covers many areas of our lives. With chronic pain, education is necessary to find the right treatment for our condition. With children, we should be involved in their education. This can involve homework. I disagree with homework, but I do my part to torment my children.

It is also useful to know about other peoples, races and religions. When we are dealing with foster children and their parents, it is necessary to try to understand where they are coming from; why they did what they did. We then know what we have to do to help their children overcome what was done to them.

Provide a safe home environment for our children.

One thing I have realized with the 130+ children is, it is paramount that we provide a safe environment for them. A home not full of physical, mental or sexual violence. A home where people don't commit suicide. A home where everyone feels safe. A harmonious home.

Dealing with pain is made easier in a safe environment that is harmonious.

Build people up

Do not pull other people down. With children we should build them up, no matter how badly they appear to be behaving; no matter how badly they are doing at school; no matter how messy their bedrooms are; we should *NEVER* negatively criticize our children, call them negative names or tell them they are bad. The behavior was bad, not them. Pulling them down will fill their spirit bubbles with unhappiness and a negative charge. A person with a permanently negatively charged spirit bubble will become withdrawn, uncommunicative, disrespectful and difficult to handle and essentially deaf.

The same should be true with everyone else we come into contact as well. Why? Because pulling others down fills both the other person's and our spirit bubbles with negative emotions. For those who suffer chronic pain, a negative spirit bubble causes stress and more pain.

Nagging

Nobody enjoys being nagged. Adults will ignore their spouse, boss or friend who nags them and so will children. If all we do is nag, scold and reprimand, our children's behavior will become worse and they will become anxious, wondering what they will get into trouble for next. They will not be able to maintain a positive spirit bubble and in extreme situations begin to hate us.

The same is true if we are in pain and on the receiving end of nagging. We need positive spirit bubbles and nagging always has the opposite effect.

Respect

We should develop mutual respect with and for our children, and others with whom we interface, using respectful language and expecting them to follow our lead. When we feel others need chastising we should first (1) tickle our amygdala (2) take a deep breath (3) take a limbic cortical pause. This way we aren't angry and say something we'll have to apologize for later.

With pain, respect for us is necessary from those we deal with. But we also need to show respect for them because this maintains a positive spirit bubble for us.

Communication

Communicating with and getting to know our family members by spending quality time together and being approachable, is the best way to maintain positive spiritual bubbles.

Talking with our children is one of the hardest parts of being a parent, especially as they become teenagers. It is, however, the most important. The best method I have found has to do with volume –

speak quietly, don't shout and by asking open-ended questions that can't be answered with a "yes" or "no" or a shoulder shrug.

Communication and respect come together, when trying to get children to do as asked. This universal problem has no guaranteed fix. My method is the broken record. In our family, we use a chore chart, but this doesn't guarantee the chores are done. I repeat my request until they do as asked. At times, I'm overwhelmed and don't need the hassles, but I force myself, by repeating my request until they do. I then take the time and energy to praise and thank them. Then surprise, surprise their spirit bubbles begin to fill with joy.

Keeping our promises.

The Talmud teaches we should "Never promise something to a child and not give it to him, because in that way he learns to lie." I often want to give up and it can be difficult to keep a promise when your get up and go has got up and gone. Still, I must keep my promises.

Be consistent.

Being consistent can be hard when you have many children, but we must be exactly that, consistent. We should be there for them at all times and in all places. Our children should know we will always be there for them.

For example, we should treat unacceptable behavior in the same way, so that he or she doesn't think there are ways to get away with things. The same is true when praising children for good behavior. When you are in a lot of pain this is very hard, but as always, it's important we do.

Another part of consistency is when children pick on their siblings. This doesn't always mean they are being nasty; they in reality want our attention. This is always a hard thing to deal with. For them, any attention is acceptable and better than getting no attention. Being shouted out for hitting little Joey is attention. If we aren't giving them attention, they feel they must find ways to be noticed. Hurting their siblings always works, as a parent generally comes quickly when they

331

hear crying. We must always attempt to do and say positive things to all of our children. The more pain we are in the harder this is to do. Nevertheless, if we want our children to feel no pain from us, it is essential we are always filling their spirit bubble with positive attention.

Being on our children's side, especially when they get it wrong is another part of being consistent. We should teach them actions have consequences and help them through the challenging times, even when waiting for our get up and go to return.

Fight the pain for them!

When I say fight the pain, I'm suggesting nothing more than doing everything we can to ignore it. For me this involves numerous pain pills, but with them I can look for joy and in a small way forget about pain. For you, I hope it's no more than counting monkeys and taking deep breaths, which I also do, when dealing with our personal chaos.

With children, we can find something positive that our child has done and praise them for doing that, instead of shouting and complaining about whatever they did wrong. The first causes joy, the second pain. There are no pain pills to overcome this hurt. If the pain isn't physical, but mental, spiritual or emotional there are medications available to help, but we still have to make a choice to be positive.

Yet another flat tire

Another experience when I could have told my little angel, LLO9, to be quiet, etc. occurred in relation to the never-ending flat tire fiasco. My record is 5 flat tires within one hour on one trip. This day I had one with an air leak. The rear driver side tire had a small hole somewhere, which was eluding me. I broke my air compressor trying to blow it up and limped to the nearest gas station and paid the offensive amount of $1 for air.

We then went to the store. As she walked past the rear of the car, LLOL9 turned and said, "I can hear air coming out of the tire." I listened and said I couldn't. She insisted she could and, pointing to a spot on the tire, said it was coming from "this hole." I checked and sure enough, there was a hole exactly where she was pointing and I could hear the air coming out of it.

I carry a tire repair kit and have become expert at putting plugs in. I plugged the tire and it stayed up. I have a miraculous story I can and have shared with others and with her when she gets older. I could have told her she was being stupid and gone into the store. I would then have returned to the car to find the tire totally flat and been very upset. LLOL9 would also have been upset and possibly behaved badly while we were in the store because of my poor behavior. She would have had the right to be badly behaved, but I probably would not have been able to accept that she had the right for very long.

Finding the negative is easy

I know how easy it is to find the pain, the negative, but think about the fact that we are building painful memories both for ourselves and the others we are experiencing the event with.

This proves, for us, love does indeed think evil. At least that sort of love does. We will often find we have to force ourselves to be positive and find joy. We have the choices to say nice things about ourselves and others and find the positive in all situations. This is a wonderful and truly copacetic choice to make.

This, of course, will not change the fact that, if our 7-year-old somehow finds and drinks a caffeinated soda, we will still be trying to scrape her off the ceiling at midnight.

The idea at the end of the book

We are now at the end of the book. Unlike the wonderful children's book Sesame Street © children's book, "There's A Monster At The End Of This Book." there is no monster here. What is here is a final suggestion

The first part is to accept that it (whatever your objective or goal is) may well be too large to achieve in one go and this is all right. Your objective may be to not swear ever again, but you have being doing so for so long you don't think you'll succeed. Chop it up into goals and tasks you feel you can handle. I helped someone do this by having him set the goal of not swearing in the morning. He considered he was successful if by 11am, he hadn't sworn, that day was a success. If he swore during the rest of the day, he wasn't failing. He would then move the target to 12pm. After moving the target several times, he was at bedtime and had not sworn all day. It took several days to reach the first target and time to reach each subsequent target, but he succeeded. He no longer swears

Any goal can be achieved using this method. Reach the first target and don't worry about anything else. In the example of swearing; cursing before 4pm was tolerable; when the goal was to reach 11am without swearing. Once the goal was 5pm, it was no longer good enough, but it didn't matter too much, because we will reach the goal tomorrow. As long as we ensure we do all we can to achieve the goal tomorrow, then we will succeed.

My mission statement

Even though I can only do a little of what I used to be able to, I find joy in what I can do. I try my best not to complain and fill my spirit bubble with joy. I will find humor and laugh more than ever. Unhappiness is the opposite of joy. I will have an attitude of gratitude. I will do all I can not to complain. I will avoid sorrow and grief, so when I've lost my get up and go, I'll wait until it returns. I **will** fill my spirit bubble with empathy. I **will not** shout. I **will** fight pain at every place it shows up and I **will** find joy, no matter what! I will never be a zounderkite. My spirit bubble will be filled with joy and happiness. And if I fail I'll pick myself up, take a deep breath, dust myself off and start all over again every time.

When fighting pain finding joy
Remember it is
THE pain,
not <u>my</u> pain

Pain does not own or define me
I do not own it.

It is what it is, bit it is not mine!

This being the information age, it's easy to contact me. You can join in my blog at
www.DavidAlanGray.com
Or email me at dave@DavidAlanGray.com

David Alan Gray lives in Southern Idaho with his wife, Ann. They are the parents of nine children, five of whom are still living at home. Born in England, he built a career as a computer consultant. He has worked for airlines, banks, government agencies, chemical producers, utility companies and in the insurance industry. He has also had his own IT business.

His career has taken the family from the North East of England to New York and Dallas before they settled in the Rocky Mountains. David and his family enjoy traveling and exploring in the great outdoors. The family has three dogs, a cat and a hedgehog, who all contribute to the general mayhem. David insists they are not his pets, but his wife and kids would disagree.